DATE DUE

MAY 1 8 1996	
DEC 2 0 1996	
APR 1 1 1999	
MAY 1 0 1999	
OCT 1 1 1999	
APR 1 7 2001	
GAYLORD	PRINTED IN U.S.A.

Childhood Sexual Abuse
and the Construction of Identity

Childhood Sexual Abuse and the Construction of Identity

Healing Sylvia

Michele L. Davies

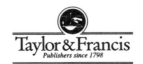

Taylor & Francis
Publishers since 1798

UK   Taylor & Francis Ltd, 4 John St., London WC1N 2ET
USA   Taylor & Francis Inc., 1900 Frost Road, Suite 101, Bristol, PA 19007

First published 1995

A Catalogue Record for this book is available from the British Library

ISBN 0 7484 0175 X
ISBN 0 7484 0176 8 pbk

Library of Congress Cataloging-in-Publication Data are available on request

Typeset in 11/13pt ITC Garamond
by Solidus (Bristol) Limited

Printed in Great Britain by Biddles Ltd, Guildford and King's Lynn on paper which has a specified pH value on final paper manufacture of not less than 7.5 and is therefore 'acid free'.

Contents

Preface

This study consists of a detailed critical examination of an account of 'incest and of healing' written by a 'survivor' of childhood sexual abuse. It is a project inspired by my rejection of the ever increasing tendency within some forms of social science to treat 'personal experience' as pre-given and foundational. As will become evident over the course of this study I find such projects not only analytically unconvincing, but also politically dangerous. I suggest that neither of these features is conducive to the production of good social science.

By contrast, my aim within this study is to analyse some of the linguistic and cultural resources used in the production of 'personal experience'. The aim of this project is to show how supposedly 'private' or psychological experiences are fundamentally connected to the social and cultural domain.

As the findings of this study indicate, this task is extremely important because it provides insight into how people negotiate responsibility and allocate blame, specifically in relation to the issue of childhood sexual abuse. It is through an analysis of these processes that this study offers critical insight into one of the most complex problems facing us in contemporary society.

Acknowledgments

I should like to thank Dr Martyn Hammersley for his valuable and consistent supervision of my PhD research on which this book is grounded. In addition, I take this opportunity to thank a multitude of other people who have expressed an interest in my work over the last few years, Jo Campling for her help in guiding *Healing Sylvia* to publication, Sylvia Fraser, Virago Press, Sterling Lord Literistic Inc. for their permission to quote from *My Father's House* and the Design and Artists Copyright Society for granting a copyright licence for Picasso's *Girl in Front of a Mirror* (front cover reproduction).

On a more personal note I should like to thank my mum and dad for providing me with the best start in life that anyone could ever have asked for and for giving me the opportunities that they themselves never had. The love, care, friendship and dedication that they have always shown me cannot be matched. So thank you, mum and dad. And Nick Crossley, my husband, my best friend. You have been an inspiration to me; your loyalty, your love, your enthusiasm, your intellect. I would like to thank you, Nick, for sharing them with me.

Chapter 1

Introduction:
The Worldliness of Subjectivity

In recent years within the social sciences, and within society more generally, there has been a great deal of emphasis on, and a celebration of, 'personal experience'. We are continually informed of the importance of discovering and affirming 'ourselves'; of the necessity of listening to and 'hearing' the 'voices' of subordinate and underprivileged groups. One area in which particular weight has been placed upon appeals to 'voices' and personal subjectivity is in (feminist) writing on childhood sexual abuse. In this first chapter, I will provide some of the historical background relating to the issue of childhood sexual abuse and chart some of the factors leading to an emphasis on the importance of personal experience. My main aim is to highlight some of the practical and theoretical problems associated with the way in which 'personal experience' has been conceptualized. Having pointed towards some of these problems I suggest an alternative perspective, which, I argue, provides a more sound academic and political base.

Childhood Sexual Abuse and Women's Experience

At the end of the last century, in his treatment of women 'hysteric' patients in Vienna, Freud found a substantial number of them reporting memories of coercive and traumatic sexual experiences with their fathers and other male, adult relatives.[1] Armed with this finding, Freud, in his 1896 paper *The Etiology of Hysteria*, set out his theory for an understanding of hysteria, now known as the 'seduction theory'. In this paper Freud's tone is compassionate. He asks: 'Poor child, what have they done to you?' (Freud, 1896). However, he was soon to retract this theory and to replace it with his newly developing theory of 'infantile sexuality' which entailed a quite different picture of 'sexual abuse'. In 1897, for example, Freud wrote to Fliess concerning his women patients who spoke of having been seduced by their fathers: 'I no longer believe in my *neurotica* (Freud to Fliess, 21 September 1897, quoted in Clark, 1980, p. 161). Here we have the replacement of the original seduction theory with that of his theory of 'infantile sexuality' which attributed unconscious drives and desires to infants and children. This theory was set forth in Freud's *Introductory Lectures* where he states that stories of childhood seduction in which the father figures as the seducer often involve an 'imaginary accusation' on the part of the patient. The upshot of this theory is that many victims experiences of paternal incest have been seen as the product of fantasies on the part of the patient.

Masson has subsequently publicized and criticized Freud's abandonment of the original theory, in *The Assault on Truth: Freud's Suppression of the Seduction Theory* (Masson, 1984a). This book derives from Masson's research on the origins of psychoanalysis in Freud's personal papers. During the course of this research, Masson found discrepancies between the original and published volumes of correspondence which led him to the conclusion that Freud had suppressed the extent of his knowledge of child seduction in order to protect his standing as a respectable member of the scientific community. However, as the subsequent Malcolm–Masson controversy has made clear (see Malcolm, 1983, 1984; Masson, 1984b; Scott, 1984), this claim is contentious. Scott, for example, has argued that Freud's theory of infantile sexuality got him into much greater difficulty than the original seduction theory had done (Scott, 1988, p. 90).

Nevertheless, in recent years, Freud's abandonment of the original seduction theory has often been taken as evidence of his contempt for women and children. While I would be reluctant to endorse this opinion, I do believe that the theory of infantile sexuality has had crucial implications for the widespread denial of the issue of child sexual abuse during much of the twentieth century. Indeed, until the advent of the Women's Liberation Movement of the late 1960s, an atmosphere of moral condemnation of victims who made such claims prevailed. Bender and Blau's 'findings' in their study of sexually abused children is not atypical. Their conclusion was as follows:

> These children undoubtedly do not deserve completely the cloak of innocence with which they have been endowed ... in some cases the child assumed an active role in initiating the relationship ... it is true that the child often rationalised with excuses of fear of physical harm or the enticement of gifts, but

there were obviously secondary reasons ... these children were distinguished as unusually charming and attractive.... Thus ... we might have frequently considered the possibility that the child might have been the actual seducer, than the one innocently seduced. (Bender and Blau, 1937, p. 509)

In the late 1960s, however, the Women's Liberation Movement set a different tone for the treatment of the issue of child sexual abuse. Feminism encouraged the development of women as a group with their own collective consciousness, advocating the woman's right to control over her own body. Issues of rape and domestic violence were no longer to be seen as individual, personal issues, but as *socio-political* issues. For example, the subtitle of Brownmiller's classic *Against Our Will* is 'Men, Women and Rape ... a conscious process of intimidation by which *all* men keep *all* women in a state of fear' (Brownmiller, 1975). The Women's Shelter Movement, initiated by Erin Pizzey in the early 1970s, similarly identified the increasing prevalence of incest and child sexual abuse in physically abusive families. This sort of consciousness-raising enabled victims of sexual abuse to verbalize and write about their experiences in a much more supportive atmosphere.

Written, autobiographical accounts of experiences of sexual abuse began to appear during the late 1960s, but they gained further ground in the late 1970s. They include: Maya Angelou's *I Know Why the Caged Bird Sings* (1969); Louise Armstrong's edited collection *A Speak-out on Incest* (Armstrong, 1978), containing 26 contributions by women who were sexually abused as children; *Father's Days* (Brady, 1979), 'a true story of incest'; Charlotte Vale Allen's *Personal Memoir* (Vale Allen, 1980); *I Never Told Anyone* (Bass and Thornton, 1983); *Father–Daughter Rape* (Ward, 1984), containing personal accounts of nine Australian women. In all of these accounts, the aim was to represent the reality of child sexual abuse from the victim's point of view, to guide the public's understanding of the 'real' nature of child sexual abuse.

These accounts are analogous to other types of 'coming-out' stories in that they address the issues of what it means to be a sexually abused child, of how such abuse figures over the course of one's life, of what it means to 'come out', to 'tell' one's story. They are accounts of the processes involved in female victims becoming conscious of themselves as sexually abused individuals, of accepting and affirming that identity. The narratives are committed to making visible the realities of the life of the sexually abused child.

This process of rendering 'visible' is made possible through the 'power of words'. In Berger's terms:

> To break the silence of events, to speak of experience however bitter or lacerating, to put into words, is to discover the hope that those words may be heard, and that when heard, the events will be judged. (Berger, 1988, p. 251)

It is in this sense that such first-person accounts are explicitly committed to the political importance of writing and reading strategies for the creation of identity, community and political solidarity (Martin, 1988, p. 80). Telling, writing and reading such accounts are linked to the important task of countering representations that have made women and children silent, invisible, deviant, perverse, aberrant or marginal. Such storytelling is thus part of the larger struggle for self-determination among oppressed and silent groups. This is evident, for example, in Vale Allen's account (1980), where she suggests that if women and girls have a stronger consciousness of the reality of sexual abuse, if they are able to communicate about experiences of the injustices perpetrated against them, then they can move some way towards the prevention of child sexual abuse. Bass and Thornton (1983) similarly highlight the important role of first-person accounts for the process of consciousness raising and education of the general public with regard to the incidence of child sexual abuse. Similarly, Ward (1984) ends her book with a 'Coda for Action', giving a theoretical statement on the nature of incest:

> The incestuous family is a microcosmic paradigm of the rape ideology which operates in the macrocosm of society. In the incestuous family, we find the most powerless of females, a girl-child, has become the sexual possession of the father, the king in his castle lording it over his concubine. (Ward, 1984, p. 193)

Here we see an implicit reference to the feminist slogan 'the personal is political'. The experiences of the individual female represent, and are in no way separable from, the patriarchal context of society. It is evident, then, that these feminist autobiographical accounts, emerging out of the climate of the late 1960s, draw on Marxist-socialist analysis of the nature of oppression. Here, the inequalities and repression suffered by women are seen as intertwined with inequalities suffered by the working class. Both are seen as a product of the material, economic and social inequalities that exist in a capitalist culture.

However, the 'profile' of events documented within these earlier accounts has not been sustained within more contemporary accounts, which are influenced by 'healing strategies'.[2] In a recent article, Kitzinger (1992) points to academic textbooks, journals, pop-psychology and self-help manuals as indicative of this movement. Amongst such self-help manuals, she cites: *Reclaiming Our Lives: Adult Survivors of Incest* (Poston and Lisbon, 1989); *The Healing Way: Adult Recovery from Childhood Sexual Abuse* (Kunzman, 1990); and *Reach for the Rainbow: Advanced Healing for Survivors of Sexual Abuse* (Finney, 1990). Another such account is Linda Sanford's *Strong in the Broken Places – Overcoming the Trauma of Childhood Abuse* (Sanford, 1991). Kitzinger does not, however, include first-person accounts as part of this movement.

During the course of my research, I have found, perhaps not surprisingly, that the very same movement towards strategies of 'healing' is evident in relation to autobiographical accounts of childhood sexual abuse. Indicative examples include: Sylvia Fraser's *My Father's House: A Memoir of Incest and of Healing* (1989); Jacqueline Spring's *Cry Hard and Swim – The Story of an Incest Survivor* (1987) and Cathy Anne Matthews's *Breaking Through – No Longer a Victim of Child Abuse* (1990). The important point to note about these contemporary accounts is that they present a rather different 'profile' of the issue of childhood sexual abuse from that available within some of the earlier accounts just discussed. I will return to this issue later. For the time being, however, it is sufficient to point out that the autobiographical accounts appearing during the late 1960s/early 1970s, and those appearing during the 1980s, draw on different resources which significantly affect the portrayal both of the issue of childhood sexual abuse, and also of the 'personal experience' of such an event.

It is important to note here that the conception of 'personal experience', which is evident in some of the later autobiographical accounts, is more akin to the perspective of so-called 'radical' or 'cultural' feminism whereas earlier accounts are largely based within the perspective of 'socialist' feminism. This distinction is very important. For example, for some 'radical' or 'cultural' feminists, the concept of 'experience' or 'subjectivity' is seen as a 'natural' or ideal state – a state that enlightened or emancipated Woman will aspire to return to. This conception of 'experience' is based on the Romantic ideal that 'truth' and 'subjectivity' originally exist in a state of grace; untainted, virginal and natural. Like the Holy Grail, they must be 'discovered'.

This celebration of 'experience' and subjectivity is perhaps most evident in the work of 'radical' feminists such as Daly (1978) and Griffin (1982) who argue that the predominance of 'objectivity' or rationality over 'subjectivity' or emotionality is linked to the domination of the masculine over the feminine and of Culture over Nature. Their proposed solution to this problem is to reverse the emphasis and to exalt the superiority of 'feminine' values, such as caring, nurturing, relatedness, mystery and spirituality, over traditionally accepted and contrastive 'male' values (Hekman, 1990, p. 41). In *Gyn/Ecology* (1978), for example, Daly aims to create a new language whereby *real truth* can be attained, truth that depends on women's *direct* experiences, unmediated by male imagery and subsequent domination (Grant, 1987, p. 101). Female knowledge, unlike male knowledge, is based on natural connections between women and to nature itself (Daly, 1978, p. 28). French has similarly argued that the patriarchal order has privileged masculine thought which is rational, logical, exclusionary, and has devalued feminine thought which is reflective, associative and circular (French, 1985, p. 94). And Griffin has juxtaposed masculine and culture to feminine and nature, arguing that:

> What is really feared is an open door into a consciousness which leads us back to the old, ancient, infant and mother knowledge of the body, in whose depths lies another form or culture not opposed to nature but instead expressing the full power of nature and our natures. (Griffin, 1982, p. 277)

These examples highlight a number of (problematic) assumptions central to the radical feminist movement. First, there is an assumption that women have an essential nature. Second, this 'nature' is defined in terms of a closeness to the natural world. And third, it is argued that the 'nature' of a woman is vastly superior to that of a man because men are associated with culture and culture entails domination. I suggest that all of these assumptions present substantial practical and theoretical difficulties, and, as the autobiographical accounts under discussion rely, to some extent, on these assumptions, it is important to delineate more clearly the nature of such difficulties.

Essentialism and 'Subjective Experience'

In recent years there has been a growing questioning of the idea that a person's knowledge can derive purely from so-called 'private' subjective experience. Indeed, there has been radical questioning of the very notion of 'private' subjective experience. In theoretical terms, this questioning has taken place on the grounds that the acceptance of 'unmediated subjectivity' as a valid foundation for knowledge leads to a position whereby, in principle, it is possible for every person to claim that their own understanding of reality is 'merely' a 'personal' construction – a product of their own 'subjective' interpretation. This, in turn, would imply that there is an infinite number of competing truths and realities within the world. From this perspective, there are, seemingly, infinite versions of the world – as many as there are individual people. In principle, one could reach the Pirandello-like conclusion that 'it is so, if you think it is so, and the "it" which is so is only in the thinking' (Pollner, 1987, p. 46).

Of course, this theoretical problem translates into a practical and, ultimately, a political problem in the course of people's everyday interaction in the social world. If every interpretation of reality is valid in its own right (by virtue of the fact that it is grounded in 'personal experience'), then how do we choose rationally between two versions in the event of a disagreement? Harraway (1988) points out that the main problem with such 'subjective' claims to knowledge is the fact that they are 'irresponsible'. By this, she means that the authors of such claims fail to locate the grounds upon which their knowledge is based and, thus, make it very difficult for other people to challenge those claims (because they have no basis upon which to build their critique). In the same vein, Cocks provides a particularly pertinent example of such an 'irresponsible' position by drawing an analogy between the imagery used by 'cultural' feminists in the evocation of the 'nature' of Woman and women's experiences (for example, the imagery of pure instinct, nature-myths, mystical identifications with the soil, etc.), and that of Fascism. Speaking from the standpoint of a Jew growing up in Nazi Germany, Cocks argues that however radical in their intent, such feminist positions can lead to 'the most grotesque kind of politics ... [as can any] ... movement rooting itself in primordial forces – just as the most grotesque kind of politics follows from a movement rooting itself in the idea of technocratic reason' (Cocks, 1984, p. 55). This is because such images are so posed in opposition to rational thought that they can be filled with any specific content by anyone at all, with no recourse left for groups associated with those images to defend themselves against vicious interpretations by means of conceptual or logical argument. Hence, the appeal to some form of foundational 'experience' as a basis for knowledge claims:

> ... is at once *authoritarian* admitting of no further discussion, and relativist, since no individual can refute another's 'immediate' apprehension of reality. Operating at a level of assertion that admits of no further elaboration or explication, those who abandon themselves to intuition give birth to dreams (or nightmares!), not to truth. (Hawkesworth, 1989, p. 545)

It is perhaps somewhat ironic that the implications of such a position become most apparent when feminist concerns are taken as a starting point. For example, if a man is accused by a woman of rape, he can appeal to his own 'subjective experience' as a means of negating her claim to rape. Although she claims that he raped her, he did not see the event in this way. He interpreted her smile and her offer of coffee as a 'come on'. He did not see much evidence of her struggling, etc., etc. In this case, if one accepts the doctrine that 'personal experience' constitutes the basis for knowledge then one has no means of adjudicating between the differing versions of events, and thus one has no means of validating or invalidating one or the other interpretation of the event that took place.

Here, a particularly pertinent example with regard to the issue of childhood sexual abuse comes to mind. This example highlights the fact that the development of a feminist programme for understanding personal experience and subjectivity, which relies upon the 'natural' or self-evident status of such claims, is ultimately self-defeating. The example I am referring to has recently gained notoriety in the media reportage of what is known as 'False Memory Syndrome' (FMS). FMS is a theory imported from the USA which states that memories of childhood sexual abuse being produced by adult 'survivors' are induced or suggested during psychotherapy. The basis for the FMS case is:

> ...the nature of memory. Memory is not a filing cabinet but a process of reconstruction, part of the imagination and, as witnesses in court cases have discovered, it can be faulty. (Grant, 1993, *The Guardian*)

Proponents of FMS, often accused parents, have been quick to latch on to the idea that memory is 'a process of reconstruction', and this, subsequently, has formed the basis of claims that their daughters have been 'coerced', by therapists, into believing false and exaggerated stories about their past. I want to return to this issue later in this chapter, for, as will become clear, it throws up some extremely interesting (moral and political) questions with regard to my own perspective on the concept of 'mind', 'subjectivity' and 'experience'. For the time being, however, it is sufficient to note that the case of the proponents of FMS has been substantially aided by the fact that therapists have failed to make explicit the grounds and the processes upon which survivors' memories of childhood sexual abuse have been founded and subsequently formulated. In this way, survivors undergoing psychotherapy have been left wide open to attack from those who do not believe in the factual status of those memories. Because the survivor, in many cases, does not have recourse to the grounds, principles and discursive practices upon which her memory is based (as will become clear as my analysis proceeds) – and subsequently, because the survivor does not have clear-cut 'logical' grounds on which to base her claim – such claims can easily be contested as unfounded and, ultimately, as 'false'. As I will proceed to argue, however, although I agree with the theoretical underpinnings of the FMS position – i.e. that 'memory is not a filing cabinet but a process of reconstruction' – the conclusions that have been drawn from this (i.e. that survivors' memories are 'false') do not necessarily follow.

The absence of clear-cut, logical grounds, I argue, does not neces-sarily indicate falsity. Neither, however, does it indicate 'truth' – especially when wars between truth and falsity are being fought in the law courts. It is in this sense that I put forward my argument that appeals to 'personal subjectivity' – to notions of 'natural' truth, 'unmediated experience' – terms used by both 'cultural'/'radical' feminists and therapists alike are ultimately self-defeating and may result, in negative *practical* consequences such as the wholesale denial of the existence of childhood sexual abuse. Furthermore, as I now proceed to argue, the position is theoretically untenable.

The 'Worldliness' of Subjectivity

The main point to note here is that the subjectivist perspective adopted by 'cultural'/'radical' feminists suffers from overly simplistic conceptions of knowledge and truth. The upshot of this position is that Woman's experience, 'subjectivity' and, ultimately, knowledge and truth (which are supposedly based on 'personal experience'), are seen as universal, pre-given, essential, ahistorical and foundational. This, of course, flies in the face of psychological, sociological, anthropological and historical research – all suggestive of vast differences with regard to the experi-ences of women in different social, historical and cultural contexts.

It is, however, important to note that the problems associated with this conceptualization of 'personal experience' are not unique to feminism, nor do they constitute a 'new' problem. Arguments and debates over the formulation of 'personal experience', and the 'sub-jective' more generally, have a long history. As Coulter (1979) has argued, the topic of mind and subjectivity, as it has been variously pursued by sociologists, philosophers, social and cognitive psycholo-gists and theoretical linguists, has frequently appealed to some inner, foundational experience as the basis of knowledge. Academics as varied as Husserl, Mead and Freud have, according to Coulter, worked from the assumption that somewhere lurks a phenomenological residue called the 'I', some subjective, 'private' centre of consciousness, which, if only it were public, 'could explain us all' (Coulter, 1979, p. 124).

The roots for attacking such assumptions regarding the nature of mind, experience, subjectivity and consciousness can be found within the works of existential phenomenologists such as Sartre, Merleau-Ponty, Heidegger and Schutz (see Roche, 1973). In their various ways, and through their different versions of humanity's existential condition, these phenomenologists criticized the idea that knowledge could exist in pure consciousness, and indeed, the idea that 'consciousness' could exist in a 'pure', 'private' and 'subjective' form. For these philosophers, consciousness was not to be seen as some Godhead existing outside the world, but as something which is inextricably connected to the social world.

For example, Heidegger's early existentialist work *Being and Time* (1962) puts forward the view that the problem of human existence can only be adequately understood when human beings are seen as belonging, essentially *within the world*. This understanding of human existence is symbolized by the word used by Heidegger to describe the human subject, i.e. *Dasein*.[3] Sartre, the leading figure in the existentialist movement, in his early work set out to show that the human situation is characterized by a lack of permanent nature or essence and, as a result, possesses a terrifying freedom of choice. In this work he relies on a notion of the 'subjective will'. His later philosophy, however, cast in a Marxist mould, explores more fully the relationship between subjectivity and the social setting of human relationships conditioned by material scarcity (see for example, his trilogy *Les Chemins de la Liberte* (Roads to Freedom 1945–9) (Sartre 1961, 1963a, 1963b).[4] In similar terms, Merleau-Ponty, another existential phenomenologist, argued that the social world is the *homeland* of our thoughts (Merleau-Ponty, 1962, p. 25):

> Truth does not 'inhabit' only 'the inner man', or more accurately, there is no inner man, man is in the world, and only in the world does he know himself. (Merleau-Ponty, 1962, p. xi)

And:

> To return to things themselves is to return to that world which precedes knowledge, of which knowledge always *speaks*. . . . The world is there before any possible analysis of mine. . . . (Merleau-Ponty, 1962, p. x)

But what, one may ask, is this 'world' preceding knowledge? This is the world of traditions, practices, relationships, institutions and structures – it is the social world. But how does one gain access to the knowledge which this social world provides us with? One absolutely crucial factor involved in this acquisition of knowledge is language. For this reason, I now proceed to focus upon the issue of language, and the increasing recognition within the social sciences of the critical role played by language in gaining an understanding of the *social* nature of human knowledge.

Over the last 30 years or so, there has been a sustained attack on the assumption that language somehow corresponds to, or can be taken as 'standing for' or as 'representative' of, states of affairs within the 'outer' social world or the 'inner' psychic world. The thrust of this attack derives mainly from the school of thought known as conceptual analysis – a general label which can be used to describe the work of Wittgenstein (1953), Ryle (1949) and Austin (1962). Both Wittgenstein in *Philosophical Investigations* (1953) and Ryle in *The Concept of Mind* (1949) examined a wide array of psychological and cognitive concepts such as 'beliefs', 'thoughts', 'feelings', 'knowledge' and consciousness. They argued against the assumption that these concepts 'refer' to any form of 'inner', 'subjective' experience. Wittgenstein's argument was based on his rejection of his own early work (in *The Tractatus*) in which he believed that it was possible to 'discover' a finite set of logical and grammatical rules that would acount for the naming of certain objects by the use of certain words (commonly known as the 'picture theory' of language). In his later work (*Philosophical Investigations*), Wittgenstein rejected this possibility, arguing that it is not possible to discover the meaning of a word by appealing to abstract, logical or grammatical rules of reference. Rather, the meaning of a word can be established only by examining the context and the manner in which it is used. The 'meaning' of a word cannot be provided in abstract, but only in relation to its use in particular contexts, in the light of practical circumstances. Language, rather than being a vehicle for naming things, is an 'activity' or 'form of life' in its own right.

This philosophical perspective on language has been adopted in some forms of social psychological study such as ethnomethodology and conversation analysis (see Heritage, 1984). Both Garfinkel and Sacks, pioneers of the ethnomethodological and conversation analytic movements respectively, emphasized the importance of analysing the way in which language is used by people in the course of their everyday lives, as a means of gaining insight into the social nature of 'individual' knowledge. Especially relevant to the study of social psychology, however, is Coulter's 'social constructionist' approach to mind (see Coulter, 1973, 1979, 1983, 1989) which has brought forth the implications of Wittgenstein's later work for psychology and sociology. For example, Coulter looks at the way in which the first person pronoun 'I' is used in the course of everyday interaction. He argues that when we use the word 'I' we do not necessarily 'refer' to some 'inner' entity, or, as he puts it, to some 'elusive residuum or a kind of opaque ontological mystery' (1979, p. 121). Similarly, when we use 'subjective referents' such as 'I think', 'I believe', 'I know', 'I feel', we do not necessarily 'refer' to inner, mental processes. Rather, when people use such descriptive terms they are actually engaging in practical activities. This point will become clearer at later stages in the book when we examine in some detail how the first-person pronoun and 'subjective referents' are used in a specific account of childhood sexual abuse. As Coulter argues, people are routinely involved in assessing both their own and other people's mental states in the course of practical social life. In terms of the implications for social scientific study, this means that concepts such as 'personal experience' and 'subjectivity' should be examined in context – preferably in the practical, everyday contexts in which people commonly make use of them. Coulter calls such a project a 'semiotics of subjectivity' (Coulter, 1979, p. 155).

Harvey Sacks's (1972a, 1972b) early work was also concerned with the way in which people describe both themselves and other people. He characterized this project as the 'problem of person categorization'. Sacks's basic argument is similar to Coulter's, because he argues that the way in which we describe a person (e.g. as a 'mother', 'daughter', 'father', 'son', etc.) is not a matter of 'ostensible' reference. That is to say,' when we categorize someone as a 'mother' we do not refer to some sort of 'essential', intrinsic identity belonging to that person, just as when we use the first-person pronoun 'I' we are not referring to some 'inner' entity. Rather, when we use certain types of categories to describe people, we are actually performing practical activities. A person does not have one category which 'refers' to him/her in a logically 'correct' fashion. Rather, the way in which a person is categorized remains dependent upon the context in which the category is being applied. Hence, the interactional context is crucial to our understanding of a person's identity. Again, this will become clearer as the book proceeds because we will examine these issues of 'person categorization' in some detail. For the time being, however, it is sufficient to note that Sacks's argument is of extreme importance for social psychology because it emphasizes the fact that a person's psychological understanding of him/herself cannot be studied in isolation from the interactive, social context. As Sacks's work on person categorization provides a crucial backdrop to this study, further details concerning his work are given in Appendix A.

Recapturing the 'Worldliness' of Subjectivity

All of the researchers just mentioned share in common the fact that they are attempting, in various ways, to retrieve the 'cultural work' that goes into the production of 'subjective' and 'personal' experience. This 'cultural work' is what I refer to when I talk of the 'worldliness' of subjectivity. Subjectivity, and the seemingly 'subjective' components and processes that go with it, such as 'self', 'identity', 'memory', 'attention', 'feeling', 'emotion' etc. do not exist in a vacuum. Rather, they are a product of cultural and discursive factors. In other words, they are essentially grounded within a cultural world. It is this world – the world of language, practices, institutions and so on – that some 'radical'/ 'cultural' feminists, conceiving of 'personal experience' as essential and foundational, fail to take into consideration.

However, it is important to note that this failure is not surprising. Most of us, in our practical orientation to the everyday world, are not aware of the fact that our actions, thoughts, feelings, indeed, our very 'selves' and our supposedly 'personal' identities, are totally enmeshed in the matrix of a social and cultural world. Our engagement within the world leads us to a radical 'forgetting' of the grounds on which our behaviour is based. This 'forgetting' is the product of years of training, socialization and, thus, institutionalization into the world in which we live our daily lives. Like any long-term relationship, each person's relationship with the world is subject to a radical 'taking-for-grantedness'. We forget where we are in the relationship. We forget where we came from. We forget where we are going to. The other, in this case the cultural world in all its various guises, is always there for us. It is always with us, it is always present. Never absent, we cannot conceive of its absence. Thus, as in all forms of 'taking-for granted', the 'work' that has gone into the relationship in the past, the way in which we got to where we are now, the 'work' that both 'I' and 'You' routinely perform to maintain the relationship – the 'work' that prevents a radical breakdown – has indeed become 'routine'. Our practices have become invisible. It is this invisibility of cultural practices that leads us to believe in the monadic individual, the 'core' self, the 'essentially subjective' – and thus, in the ultimate possibility of 'discovering' our 'true' selves – our selves that lie somewhere deep 'within' us, our true selves that possess the ultimate Truth.

The way in which cultural practices are rendered invisible was highlighted in a classic study performed by Garfinkel, Livingstone and Lynch (1981). This study analysed how astronomers at the Steward Observatory 'discovered' an optical pulsar. Contrary to the image of 'independent discovery' that is often put forward in scientific studies, Garfinkel *et al.* suggest that the 'Galilean pulsar' is a 'cultural object' which is constructed through the scientific practices employed by the astronomers. The relation between the pulsar and the activities through which it is detected is akin to the relation between the potter's hand and the pot it shapes (Garfinkel, Livingstone and Lynch, 1981, p. 137): the existence of the pulsar is 'intertwined' with the embodied practices through which it is addressed and sought out. However, although the pulsar and its discovery are 'intertwined' with the actual practices employed by the astronomers, these practices are disattended over the course of discovery, and in journal accounts of that discovery. The 'forgetting' of these practices enables scientists to construct an image of 'discovery' in which the pulsar is seen as a 'natural object' which exists independently of the scientists' methodological and theoretical framework.

For my purposes, however, the important point to make clear about this study is that Garfinkel *et al.* demonstrated the possibility of retrieving these 'forgotten' practices. They managed to make visible the 'work of fact production in flight'. The aim of the study was to reveal some of the cultural practices involved in the genesis of knowledge. This task is directly analogous to my own aim within this study, albeit applied to a different domain of knowledge. I will now proceed to expand on the area of knowledge which this book takes as its subject-matter.

The focus of this study, as the title suggests, is the relationship between childhood sexual abuse and identity. My use of the word 'identity' is intended to refer to a whole range of supposedly 'subjective' processes such as memory, emotion, beliefs etc. – processes which are commonly seen as contributing to an individual's personality. As my argument has so far foreclosed, however, I do not intend to 'return' to some 'inner', subjective, private experience as a means of accessing this domain of knowledge. Rather, my aim will be to examine how 'personal experience' of 'memories', 'beliefs' and 'identities' relating specifically to the issue of childhood sexual abuse can be located within the 'public' domain of cultural, discursive and institutional practices. This has the implication that knowledge claims are rendered 'responsible', i.e. publicly accountable, as opposed to the 'irresponsible', i.e. non-publicly accountable knowledge claims of the advocate of 'private' experiential truth.

Public Accountability and False Memory Syndrome (FMS)

On a final note in this chapter, it is pertinent to point out that my emphasis on the importance of public accountability and the practical implications of such accountability is particularly resonant in light of the contemporary problem of FMS. As I have already suggested, survivors' appeals to memories lying deep within their psyche as the basis of their claims that they were sexually abused as children are proving to be ultimately self-defeating in terms of public recognition of the occurrence of childhood sexual abuse. This is because proponents of FMS can point to the 'survivors' ' lack of logical grounds for making such claims, and this, in a court of law, often translates into a powerful argument against accepting the truth of a woman's accusation.

The proponents of FMS, drawing on the idea that memory is not a filing cabinet but 'a process of reconstruction', argue that vulnerable women are being induced into the belief that they were sexually abused as children by therapists using psychotherapeutic techniques such as hypnosis and psychosynthesis. Thinking from the point of view of both a social constructionist and a feminist, initially, the difficulties related to this issue threw me into something of a quandary. On the one hand, the image of memory put forward by advocates of FMS is culled from social constructionist forms of thought. A central feature of a social constructionist approach to the mind, as I have already suggested in this chapter, is an emphasis on the *way in which* different discursive and cultural practices work to produce certain images of 'mind', 'subjectivity', 'memory', etc. By highlighting the way in which such practices produce a certain vision of mental processes, one is able to demonstrate that such 'processes' are not fixed and immutable, but are, rather, changing and malleable. Moreover, on this basis, if the effects of cultural practices are in any way damaging to a particular group of persons, this position allows one to challenge and, through processes of negotiation and action, to effect a change in the identified problem. Indeed, research undertaken in the tradition of social constructionism has been particularly critical of the way in which the predominant 'psychiatric' ideology, represented by the powerful mental health industry, especially prevalent in the USA and Britain, has served to formulate the nature of certain problems. This type of approach stems from Szasz's (1961) *The Myth of*

Mental Illness and other researchers in the anti-psychiatric camp. In terms of a feminist slant to this kind of social constructionist position, Smith's (1978, 1983, 1990, 1992) work on the discursive production of femininity provides a decisively critical stance towards psychiatric formulations of experience. Kitzinger's (1988, 1992) work on the cultural production of childhood sexual abuse, and her subsequent critique of psychiatric formulations of such issues, is also of interest here.

The important point to note here, however, is that if a researcher emphasizes the way in which memory is culturally produced and, thereby, criticizes psychiatric formulations of such events, this seems to place the researcher 'on the side', so to speak, of the proponents of FMS. This, however, is not necessarily the case. As I suggested earlier, an emphasis on the social and discursive constitution of memory does not imply that such 'memories' are necessarily 'false' – as the proponents of FMS conclude. Having looked at the way in which all subjectivity, personhood, identity and so on can be seen as belonging essentially 'within the world' (via existential phenomenologists such as Sartre, Heidegger, Merleau-Ponty and conceptual analysts such as Wittgenstein and Ryle), we should now be in a position to see why this conclusion does not follow.

This is because everything pertaining to the world of *human* life, everything that has relevance for human beings, 'belongs' to and is constructed by discursive and cultural practices. To be a human being and to live as a human being implies a total enmeshing in the matrix of cultural practices. Hence, if it is the case that memories of childhood sexual abuse are 'false' *by virtue* of the fact that they are based on cultural practices (such as psychotherapeutic practices), then it must also be the case that every other aspect of reality based on any form of cultural practice must also be false. The implications of the FMS position, then, must be that all of human life is 'false', and that, ultimately, there is no truth. Moreover, it is important to note that proponents of FMS who contest the truth of survivors' experiential claims *on the basis* of the fact that these claims are influenced by cultural practices, ultimately betray the fact that they, like the 'cultural'/'radical' feminists, presuppose the possibility of a 'naïve', 'natural', 'untainted' and 'unmediated' 'experiential truth' – truth that is *not* based on cultural practices.

As my argument has foreclosed, however, I dispute this possibility. I dispute the idea that an individual has 'privileged access' to an 'inner truth'. I dispute the idea that memory consists of a set of inner workings – a filing cabinet in which information is stored. I dispute the idea that identity and personality consist of some set of innate, unique qualities that, again, only the individual concerned has access to. My alternative claim is that 'truth', 'memory' and 'identity' are all unique features of human social life – and, as such, they are subject to discursive, cultural practices. In other words, they live in a 'public', intersubjective domain, as opposed to a 'private', subjective domain. In this sense, the 'nature' of these phenomena is not an idiosyncratic feature of the individual's subjectivity but is, rather, intrinsic to the culture in which the individual belongs.

My investigation of the nature of such phenomena therefore – here, with specific reference to the issue of childhood sexual abuse and its impact on identity – suggests that a 'new' way forward is required. This involves an analysis of the way in which such events are constructed. This programme has already begun in the various fields of ethnomethodology, historical research in the Foucauldian tradition and poststructuralist feminist work (e.g. Cocks, 1984; Scott, 1986, 1991; Hawkesworth, 1989; Butler, 1990; Hekman, 1990). The research emerging from these traditions of thought shares a common theme – namely, an attempt to deconstruct categories of 'experience' and to examine the relationships between experience, knowledge and power. In all of this there is a concern to locate the 'public' grounds on which 'personal' phenomena are based. Ultimately, I suggest that the aim of such research is to locate the grounds on which a *critical* stance towards a given phenomenon can be taken. By locating 'experience' within the space of public, discursive formations – and by deconstructing those categories – the ground is laid for possible and potential reconstructions.

Conclusion

In this chapter, my aim has been to provide an alternative formulation of 'subjectivity' and 'personal experience' to that available within some forms of feminist inquiry. I have argued that such inquiries encounter many theoretical and practical difficulties because they fail to take into account the essentially public dimension of experiential and subjective categories. As a means of providing an alternative to this approach, I have pointed towards various approaches which move away from the idea that subjectivity consists of an 'inner', 'mental' phenomenon, or that meaning and interpretation 'belong' solely to a specific individual. Rather, such phenomena are seen as 'belonging' inseparably, to the social and cultural world. Accordingly, in order to grasp the full significance of people's 'thoughts', 'feelings', 'understandings', 'experiences', 'voices' and 'points of view', we must return to an analysis of the public communicative world. In the chapters that follow, I highlight how such an approach can be applied empirically to a specific study of 'self' and 'identity'.

Notes

1. I first became interested in the issue of childhood sexual abuse when I was employed as a clinical psychologist on a reminiscence therapy/oral history project at a large psychiatric institution in London. Here, I was encouraged to 'listen to the voices' of the elderly. I did exactly that, and, as my 'clients' were mainly women, it is perhaps not surprising that I found many of them, either implicitly or explicitly, recounting traumatic experiences of childhood sexual abuse.
2. This emphasis is not confined to accounts of child sexual abuse. Open any issue of a magazine such as *Psychology Today* and one is struck by a plethora of 'healing' strategies for various 'disorders', e.g. 'healing' from eating disorders, 'healing' from 'shyness', etc.
3. The word *Dasein* means 'being-in-the-world'. Literally translated, as can be shown by breaking the word with a hyphen to display its etymological construction ('Da-sein'), it is 'Being-there' (Heidegger, 1962, p. 27).
4. A similar development can be seen in the existentialist Simone de Beauvoir's work, especially in the second volume of her autobiography *La Force de l'Age* (The Prime of Life, 1965). Over the first half of the narrative de Beauvoir establishes both herself and Sartre (her friend and lover) as independent, free, and surrounded by almost unlimited choices. With the onset of the Second World War, however, limitations and restrictions are imposed upon de Beauvoir (mainly expressed in her enforced separation from Sartre), which force her to revise her philosophy of human freedom (here, I owe thanks to Nick Crossley for our discussions regarding the relationship between Sartre's and de Beauvoir's increasingly politicized philosophy – see Crossley, 1994). The publication of de Beauvoir's third volume of autobiography *La Force des Choses* (The Force of Circumstance, 1968) highlights her move towards Marxist philosophy. This part of the autobiography had a 'mixed reception'. For example, a review in England berated it for its political stance and 'lack of humour' (Okley, 1986, p. xvii).

Chapter 2

Childhood Sexual Abuse and Autobiographical Materials

In Chapter 1 I argued that 'personal experience', 'mind', 'subjectivity', etc., are constituted through cultural and discursive practices. This, I suggested, has implications for the way in which certain events and experiences are interpreted. In particular, I proposed to examine the issue of survivors' experiences of childhood sexual abuse from this discursive standpoint. These 'experiential' accounts, I suggested, embody a historical shift. Published accounts of experiences of childhood sexual abuse appearing during the late 1960s/70s are largely influenced by a socialist feminist perspective. By some contrast, accounts being published during the 1980s/90s owe more to a 'cultural'/ 'radical' feminist perspective. Whereas the socialist feminist perspective emphasizes the material, social and economic basis on which 'experience' and subjectivity is based, the same cannot be said of the 'radical'/ 'cultural' feminist perspective. Rather, the latter perspective advocates a 'return' to a 'subjective experience' that is pre-cultural, and, to some extent, independent from the material basis of society. In this sense, the 'cultural'/'radical' feminist perspective is akin to certain psychiatric models of experience which similarly presuppose a 'consciousness' or 'psyche' that is independent of cultural practices. The analogy, indeed, the cross-over between the 'radical'/'cultural' feminist position and the psychiatric position becomes most evident when one considers the 'healing' strategies that both perspectives advocate for 'survivors' of childhood sexual abuse.

In this chapter I concentrate on one particular autobiographical account – a relatively recent account written by Sylvia Fraser, entitled *My Father's House – A Memoir of Incest and of Healing* (1989). I take this account as a particularly revealing instance of the wider historical shift characterized above. For this reason, I propose to provide a detailed analysis of Fraser's account over the course of this study.

Sylvia Fraser's *My Father's House* is one of the best known autobiographical accounts of childhood sexual abuse. In Bagley and King's terms: 'Of all the other personal accounts of sexual abuse in childhood, Sylvia Fraser's . . . is the most remarkable' (Bagley and King, 1990, p. 18). Somewhat interestingly, one reviewer of Fraser's text has interpreted it as representative of the socialist feminist perspective so characteristic of earlier autobiographical accounts published in the late 1960s/70s. In an article in *New Statesman and Society*, Vincent suggests that Fraser has:

> . . . the form to take a crack at it (the truth) without embellishing her narrative with little shocks and horrors that *separate the psychology she shares with all other women from the pathology of her father's house.* (Vincent, 1989, p. 43)

In other words, Vincent suggests that Fraser's account, like earlier socialist feminist-inspired accounts, attempts to dissolve the boundaries between the 'private' and the 'public' and to locate the 'personal' within the grounds of the 'political', i.e. within the context of cultural practices and power relationships. Such an interpretation of Fraser's text can be attributed to a number of factors. First, Fraser has an established reputation as a 'feminist' writer (largely due to the publication of her feminist novel *Pandora* in 1972). Indeed, Fraser emphasizes this part of her identity at various stages throughout *My Father's House*. Second, *My Father's House* is published under a feminist imprint, namely Virago. And third, as will become evident over the course of the subsequent chapters, it is possible to interpret the text in this way by selectively emphasizing certain parts of Fraser's text. As I will proceed to argue, however, Fraser's text can only be interpreted in this way by omitting large sections of the book. Thus, Vincent only discusses the first two sections of Fraser's text, thereby omitting any reference to, or consideration of, the final four sections (i.e. over half of the text). As will become increasingly evident, these sections are influenced by a very different model of events from that available within the first part of the text. This has important practical implications for the issue of childhood sexual abuse.

The 'model' of events that I am referring to here is one culled from what can be called the 'healing' discourse – a discourse shared, as I have already suggested, by the 'cultural'/'radical' feminists and some forms of psychiatry. From within this discourse, a person's experiential or personal 'truth' is not related to a cultural or 'political' reality in the same way as is the case from within the socialist feminist discourse. Rather, to reiterate, a 'personal' or experiential truth from within the 'healing' discourse is something unique and idiosyncratic to the individual concerned. This is the predominant image of truth, knowledge and reality evident in Fraser's book. Evidence of this can be seen from the way in which the majority of reviewers have responded to *My Father's House*. For example, there has been a great deal of emphasis on the capacity of 'personal experience' to 'express' the 'truth'. The book has been described as containing 'the bright clear edge of truth . . .' (Vincent, 1989, p. 44); it is a 'remarkable testimony . . .' (Sayer, 1989, p. 23). Further, it is a book which contains *the personal truth of her own abuse . . .* (Bagley and King, 1990, p. 20). It is described as *her story* (Mitchell, 1988). Here, I am drawing attention to the fact that Sylvia Fraser's 'story', her 'truth', is seen as 'belonging', almost exclusively, to her. In this sense, 'the truth' of her childhood appears as something of a 'personal possession'.

This is further indicated by the fact that reviewers' reports of *My Father's House* become very personal, repeatedly alluding to Fraser's 'personal qualities'. For example, '*My Father's House* . . . is told with compassion and honesty' (Mackay, 1987, p. 3); 'her continuing candour is exemplary' (Kirkus Reviews, 1988, p. 56); The book is characterized as 'sensitive' and 'courageous'; the story is told 'with eloquence, compassion and almost unbearable candour . . .' (Mitchell, 1988); it is 'A beautifully written, heart-wrenching and ultimately healing story by an amazing and courageous woman' (Atwood, cited on the cover of Fraser, 1989); it has 'tremendous power, candour and eloquence . . . a terrible account of a woman's coming of age and a lyric story of love and forgiveness' (cited on the cover of Fraser, 1989) and; 'The final chapter of this book is extraordinary, beautiful and lyrical, like a soliloquy culminating an opera by Janecek' (Bagley and King, 1990, p. 21).

Here, then, is an overwhelming picture of reviewers commending Fraser for her laudable 'personal qualities'; for her 'candour' and her 'honesty' – both qualities which, ultimately, lead to her capacity for 'love and forgiveness'. My main point of emphasis, however, is the way in which such qualities are personalized and 'attached' to Sylvia Fraser. The text is seen as representative of Fraser's personal qualities, in much the same way as it is seen as representative of her 'personal truth'. However, just as I have argued that 'personal truth' does not exist in a vacuum, detached from discursive and cultural practices, so the same argument applies to 'personal qualities'. Fraser's capacity for 'love and forgiveness', a capacity much applauded by the reviewers, does not emerge from nowhere. As I will proceed to argue, Fraser's capacity for love and forgiveness and, moreover, her belief in the *necessity* for love and forgiveness, emerges from her use of a specific discursive practice as a means of making sense of her experience.

It is important to emphasize that I am not in any way denying the fact that Sylvia Fraser is 'honest', that she displays 'candour' or that she has an extensive capacity for love and forgiveness. Here, it may be useful to recall my critique of the proponents of FMS set forth in Chapter 1. The fact that memories are based on cultural practices does not necessarily imply that those memories are 'false'. Similarly, the fact that Fraser's 'amazing' capacity for love and forgiveness is based on cultural practices does not necessarily mean that she is not capable of such capacities. The point is, however, that such a capacity is not merely the product of her own 'unique' and idiosyncratic personality. It is, rather, a capacity that she has, in some way, learned, and that has, thereby, become a feature of her personality as expressed in her autobiography. That is to say, a capacity for love and forgiveness develops in accordance with certain norms and conventions, and cannot be reduced to the individual. It is a capacity that is grounded in certain cultural practices and, as such, has effects extending far beyond the realm of the individual. It is for this reason that I believe it is of the utmost importance to examine the grounds of such beliefs. In the case of Sylvia Fraser, I suggest that her capacity for love and forgiveness (as they are portrayed in her autobiography) emerge from her adoption of the 'healing discourse'. As will become evident as the analysis proceeds, the issues at stake here are wide ranging and extend far beyond the realm of the individual. These issues include social, moral and legal problems such as the allocation of blame and responsibility and, ultimately, implications for social policy with regard to the issue of childhood sexual abuse.

The 'Healing Discourse'

So far, then, I have repeatedly alluded to the fact that Fraser's 'personal experience' and, thus, *My Father's House*, is premised upon discursive practices – more specifically, upon a 'healing discourse'. What, exactly, do I mean by this? Before I elaborate on this issue I will provide a brief overview of Fraser's text.

Overview of *My Father's House*

- *Author's Note* – Statement of author's intentions; background to the text's focus and structure.
- 1 *Remembering* – Childhood years and early adolescence.
- 2 *Rescue* – Late adolescence, university years and marriage.
- 3 *Retreat* – Marriage, adultery, decline into depression and 'mental illness', divorce, death of father.
- 4 *Revelation* – Mental and physical illness, vivid dreams which serve as the source of memories of childhood sexual abuse.
- 5 *Resolution* – Retrospective analysis of parents' actions.
- 6 *Postscript* – Retrospective comments.

Over the course of my detailed, empirical examination of Fraser's text, it soon became apparent to me that the account is based on the model of psychoanalytic procedure established by Freud in his 1914 paper *Remembering, repeating and working through* (Freud, 1914, pp. 145–6). As a way of demonstrating this I will now provide a brief sketch of some of the major themes relevant to the psychoanalytic procedure. This will serve as a means by which I can highlight the comparison between the psychoanalytic model and the structure of Fraser's text. The chapters that follow will provide a more detailed analysis of this relationship and its implications.

As Freud himself pointed out, the amount of overlap between the three stages of the psychoanalytic method, recollection, repetition and working through, differs depending upon the particular case. In the case of Fraser's text the overlap is considerable. The first step, *Remembering*, is represented in the first two sections of Fraser's text *Remembering* and *Rescue*. 'Recollection' involves the method of free association whereby the patient in analysis is expected to say whatever occurs to her without censorship. This is called the *basic rule* of psychoanalysis. The rationale for this method is based on the observation that when conscious, goal-directed thinking is partly relinquished in favour of spontaneously emerging thought contents, part of the habitual defence against unconscious material can be bypassed. This unconscious material and the difficulties patients have in remembering is related to *resistances* or defence mechanisms – a process in which relevant memories and related feelings are shut off from consciousness. These mechanisms preserve the underlying, unconscious trend towards neurosis.

Through the technique of free association it is expected that the patient will remember previously forgotten experiences and situations.

The frequency and relative length of psychoanalytic sessions promotes a gradual reactivation of past emotions, fantasies, memories and thoughts, which are thus made available to the conscious ego of the patient. In the first section of Fraser's text, the defence mechanisms censoring Sylvia's thoughts as a child are made clear to the reader. This part of Fraser's text, representing the first step of the psychoanalytic procedure, comprises the focus of my Chapter 4.

The first and second steps of the psychoanalytic procedure, *Remembering and Repeating*, are represented in the third section of the text, *Retreat*. Here, further activation of past emotions, memories and thoughts is charted. Additionally, in this section the text represents the process of repetition or transference in which early warded-off tendencies and experiences are re-enacted as modified unconscious repetitions. Resistances associated with early infantile objects are transposed into the present as a new version of infantile pathogenic conflicts is unconsciously relived in the patient's efforts to free associate. This part of the text comprises the focus of my Chapter 5.

The second and third steps of the psychoanalytic procedure, *Repeating and Working Through*, are represented in the fourth section of the text, *Revelation*. Through the process of repetition, the warded-off and defensive forces that are inaccessible to change as long as they remain unconscious are made conscious. It is then important to work through the resistances and to help the patient understand what they reveal with regard to the neurosis. This entails the process of interpretation, sometimes referred too as *id interpretation*, which involves pointing out the impact of resistances on the behaviour of the patient in the past and the present. This is achieved with reference to dreams, symptoms and associations – which eventually enables the re-establishment of disrupted connections and the gaining of insight; in Fraser's terms, the 'discovery' of her truth. This section of the text will be examined in Chapter 6. The fifth section of Fraser's text, *Resolution*, and the *Postscript*, further represent the process of interpretation, a process informed by the implicit adoption of psychoanalytic insight. These sections of the text will be examined in Chapters 7 and 8.

As the subsequent chapters of this study will demonstrate, this psychoanalytic model of events has a major impact on the way in which the personal experience of the victim, namely, Sylvia Fraser, is constructed. It also, of course, has major implications for the way in which the experiences of other persons involved (e.g. the perpetrator) or implicated (e.g. the mother) in the sexually abusive events are constructed. Here, we confront issues such as the allocation of blame and the negotiation of responsibility. In the chapters that follow I highlight some of the substance of these debates with specific reference to the case of Sylvia Fraser, but also in relation to the issue of childhood sexual abuse more generally.

It is also important to bear in mind the wider historical location of the 'healing discourse', especially as it is related to the issue of childhood sexual abuse. In order to do this it is necessary to return to the starting point of this chapter, and to recall some of the details regarding the history of the child sexual abuse movement. As I have already suggested, the earlier autobiographical accounts published during the 1960s/70s produced a different picture of the relationship between the 'personal' and the 'political' from that evident in the later 1980s/90s accounts which, I argue, are largely influenced by the 'healing discourse'. As will become clear over the course of this analysis, this, in turn, results in a totally different conception of the very nature of childhood sexual abuse. Indeed, this is so much the case that it could be argued that the two discursive formations (socialist feminism on the one hand and the 'healing discourse' on the other), serve to construct entirely different 'moral profiles' of the parties involved in the event of childhood sexual abuse. These moral profiles are most apparent in terms of the different explanations and solutions to the issue of child sexual abuse offered by the two different approaches.

It is important, however, to note that these discursive formations, and the 'solutions' they put forward, do not exist in isolation from one another. Since the early feminist discourse provides the historical background for the contemporary 'healing' discourse, and since, in turn, psychoanalysis provided the historical background for the initial feminist address of the issue of childhood sexual abuse, the two discursive formations must be seen as interconnected. Indeed, as will become evident in my analysis of *My Father's House*, the early feminist discourse and the more contemporary 'healing' discourse co-exist in a continuous and mutual tension, sparring with and against each other, participating in what Bakhtin calls a 'dialogical relationship' (Bakhtin, 1981, p. 266) or what one might refer to as a 'fictive' trial. In practice, the two discursive formations continuously attempt to undercut, undermine and render irrelevant the insight provided by the opposing side; they continuously negotiate with one another. Over the course of this analysis it will be my aim to highlight the way in which such practices of negotiation are put into operation. Ultimately, this analysis will demonstrate further the way in which 'experience', 'reality' and 'truth' do not exist in some pre-given, ahistorical realm, but are, rather, based on the social and cultural practices of a given historical era.

Chapter 3

The Discursive Construction of Identity

Background

Sylvia Fraser's *My Father's House* describes the sexual abuse of the author, as a child, by her father. In order to cope with the abusive situation, Sylvia characterizes herself as having 'split into two'. Thus, from around the age of seven, she acquired an 'other self' who performed the sexual activities required of her by her father. As an adult, Sylvia originally had no recollection of these events, as she suffered from amnesia. Recovering the memory of traumatic scenes from her childhood enabled the author to progress from the experiences of mental disintegration towards a 'healed' state.

Although the actual clinical terminology of 'dual personality disorder' or 'multiple personality disorder' are not used by Fraser in order to characterize her experiences, the symptoms displayed within the text do indicate a crucial connection. This is not surprising as, in contemporary terms, the link between personality disorder and child sexual abuse is so much established that it is often taken as a foregone conclusion. This relationship was popularized in contemporary terms, in 1973, with the publication of Schreiber's *Sybil* which documents Cornelia Wilbur's (a self-styled psychoanalyst) case study of her patient 'Sybil' (Hacking, 1991a, p. 840). Moreover, in 1986 the National Institute for Mental Health survey of one hundred multiple personality disorder cases found that 97 per cent of these cases reported experiences of 'significant trauma in childhood' (Putnam *et al.*, 1986).

The American Psychiatric Association has published a series of *Diagnostic and Statistical Manuals* referred to by the acronyms *DSMII*, *DSMIII*, and *DSMIII(R)* (the R is for 'revised'). In *DSMII*, published in 1963, multiple personality disorder was not recognized as a distinct entity. With the publication of *DSMIII* in 1980, however, multiple personality disorder was specified, although the criteria and 'associated features' were somewhat narrowly defined. The revised version of *DSMIII*, published in 1987, identifies these criteria in less restrictive terms. Two centrally defined criteria are: (1) The existence within the individual of two or more distinct personalities (each with its own relatively enduring pattern of perceiving, relating to and thinking about the environment and one's self); (2) Each of these personality states at some time, and recurrently, takes full control of the individual's behaviour (*DSMIII(R)* APA, 1987, p. 106). The *DSMIII* criteria further suggest that:

> The individual personalities are nearly always quite discrepant and frequently seem to be opposites . . . [for instance] . . . 'a quiet retiring spinster' and a 'flamboyant, promiscuous bar *habitué*'. (DSMIII, APA, 1980, p. 257)

As will become clear, Fraser's text displays these definitive criteria of multiple personality disorder.

My interest in Fraser's case, however, is not to ask whether or not it 'really' is a case of multiple personality disorder. Or, for that matter, to ask whether or not multiple personality disorder 'really' exists, which, in itself, is an issue of some contention (Hacking, 1992). Rather, as should be clear by now, Fraser's text is of interest for this study in terms of the crucial issues it throws up with regard to questions of 'self', 'subjectivity', 'identity', 'consciousness', 'knowledge' and 'truth'. My aim is to examine how 'subjective' states of knowledge are produced and reproduced in practice, and, furthermore, to specify some of the social, political and moral implications of such practices. What assumptions lie behind such practices? How are 'selves' and 'identities' constructed as 'normal' or 'abnormal'; as unitary or multiple – and, again, what are the implications of such practices? These are some of the thorny, intertwined issues and interests comprising the focus for this study. Here, then, we 'return' to the 'subject' and the 'subjective', not as something that is 'inner' or 'private', but as a 'worldly' object – a cultural object that we can observe via an analysis of linguistic and discursive practices.

The Visibility of the 'Subjective'

Formulations

How, then, does the author account for her 'subjectivity', her 'identity'? In order to address this question, it is useful to draw on Garfinkel and Sacks's concept of 'formulations' – a concept which is drawn from conversation analysis. Although this concept is most frequently applied to the analysis of transcribed conversations (i.e. to oral speech), it can also be applied equally well to written accounts. Basically, formulations are characterized by the fact that at certain points within a conversation or text, a person may:

> ... treat some part of the conversation as an occasion to describe that conversation, to explain it, or characterise it, or explicate, or translate or summarise, or furnish the gist of it, or take note of its accordance with rules, or remark on its departure from rules. That is to say, a member may use some part of the conversation as an occasion to *formulate* the conversation. (Garfinkel and Sacks, 1970, pp. 350–1)

That is to say, formulations are used when a person is concerned to 'turn back' on what s/he has so far spoken or written about, in order to make explicit the meaning of the conversation or text that s/he is engaging with.

When a person does this (i.e. makes explicit the meaning of his/her previous conversation), they may also be performing a number of other (interrelated) functions. For instance, they may be *preserving* the meaning of the conversation/text so far established within the course of interaction. Such an attempt to preserve meaning is important because it enables people to maintain an element of continuity and coherence, and this is particularly significant over the course of long conversations or lengthy texts. Another function that may be performed by making explicit the meaning of the conversation/text is that of *deleting* or evading issues that may have cropped up previously, but which the speaker/author does not intend (for various reasons) to address any further. This, in turn, relates to another function that may be performed by making explicit the meaning of a conversation/text – that of *transforming* the whole significance of the previous course of inter-action. These three interrelated functions, preserving, deleting and transforming, can thus be seen as essential features of the role of formulating or making explicit the meaning of a conversation/text. This will become clearer as we examine the way in which formulations are employed in Sylvia Fraser's text in order to achieve specific objectives.

Before doing so, however, it is important to note briefly that conversation analysts have argued that formulations occur at three different but interrelated 'levels' of conversation. These 'levels' of conversation occur first at the level of 'utterance-by-utterance', by which is meant the way in which one person 'utters' or 'asks' a question and is then responded to by another person. The notion of 'utterance-by-utterance' basically refers to such sequences as 'question' and 'response'. The second 'level' of conversation in which formulations take place, according to conversation analysts, is at the level of 'topic'. This refers, somewhat self-evidently, to the actual substance or 'topic' of the conversation. And, third, formulations take place at a third 'level' of conversational organization, that of 'overall structure'. This refers to the way in which a conversation is 'summed up' or brought to an overall close. It is important to note that these 'levels' do not exist in isolation from one another. An 'orderly' conversation (or account) is one in which all three levels are integrated (Heritage and Watson, 1980, p. 251). In the analysis that follows, I will attempt to show how Fraser uses formulations at the various 'levels' of 'utterance-by-utterance', 'topic' and 'overall structure' in the organization of her text. In this way, we will gain a more concrete understanding of the way in which people use formulations in order to achieve specific practical and moral objectives.

Formulations at the Level of 'Topic'

In his analysis of telephone calls to a suicide prevention centre, Sacks discovered that formulations in conversations often occur at the opening stages of conversational encounters. Sacks called this the phenomenon of 'first-topic' analysis. For example, in telephoning a suicide prevention centre, a person is expected, in the very opening stages of his/her call, to give an explanation of the 'reason' for his/her call. In other words, they are expected to make explicit the meaning of their act. Moreover, this meaning has both practical and moral implications for the person calling the suicide prevention centre. The same observation can be made with regard to written accounts. Whether it be in the form of a 'Foreword', 'Author's Note', 'Preface' etc., in the very opening stages of the text the author is expected to provide an explanation which accounts for the text's existence.

In Fraser's account, the Author's Note can, therefore, be seen as a particularly clear example of a formulation at the level of 'first-topic' analysis. An examination of the Author's Note is revealing because it has the capacity to show the crucial role played by 'first-topic analysis' in establishing certain themes that will be relevant throughout the rest of the text. In turn, this will demonstrate how the three central properties of formulations, namely, *preservation, deletion* and *transformation*, operate within the text. The Author's Note is reproduced below for the reader's reference:

AUTHOR'S NOTE

The story I have told in this book is autobiographical. As a result of amnesia, much of it was unknown to me until three years ago. For clarity, I have used italics to indicate thoughts, feelings and experiences pieced together from recently recovered memories, and to indicate dreams. It is important to keep this device in mind while reading this book. To provide focus and structure, I have used many of the techniques of the novelist. I have also adopted fictional names and otherwise disguised persons who appear in the narrative. No attempt has been made to create full or balanced characterisations, only to portray such persons and myself as our lives relate to this difficult story. However, to my knowledge, I have not exaggerated or distorted or misrepresented the truth as I now understand it. That my father did sexually abuse me has been corroborated by outside sources. Our family secret, it appears, was not such a secret after all.

In this note, Fraser frames her account in a fashion analogous to the subjectivistic perspective characteristic of some radical feminists, outlined in Chapter 1. This is an important point because, by so doing, the author establishes a major 'topic' or 'theme' which will be preserved over the course of the whole account; namely, the foundational authority of 'personal experience' and subjectivity. For example, Fraser announces that: 'The story I have told in this book is autobiographical'. This statement builds on the subtitle of the account – 'a *memoir* of incest and of healing'.[1] Is it not the case, however, that the last two sentences of the Author's Note render my interpretation of Fraser's position as 'subjectivistic' invalid? Does she not appeal to the fact that the abuse she suffered as a child was corroborated by 'objective' sources? For the time being I merely want to point out that this statement in no way invalidates my interpretation, but in fact adds further support to it. This is because the essential point to bear in mind is the way in which Fraser constructs the *sequence* of her discovery of the truth and knowledge. I will return to discuss this point in more detail at a later stage within this chapter.

Fraser is, as I have already suggested, concerned to display the essentially 'private' nature of her knowledge. This is apparent in her frequent use of possessive pronouns such as 'my' and 'our'. She informs the reader that her aim is to 'portray such persons and *myself* as *our* lives relate to this difficult story'. When pronouns are used possessively in this way, 'personal troubles' and 'problems' are often viewed as 'owned' (Watson, 1987, p. 280). Persons 'owning' problems may be regarded as having certain rights and obligations concerning those problems, for example as regards knowledge and definition of the problem. The notion of 'possessing' problems is deeply embedded in a broad range of cultural conventions. The person who 'tells' his or her own life story is expected to have access to uniquely privileged knowledge that no one else could possibly have. It is with reference to such background expectations that the reader is likely to 'honour' Fraser's account and 'willingly suspend disbelief', bracketing his/her own judgment in favour of the author's.[2]

The possessive relationship established by Fraser towards her own knowledge performs both an inclusionary and an exclusionary function. The reader is excluded from the all-inclusive 'private' and 'privileged' knowledge of the author. In this respect, the relationship between reader and author can be said to form an 'asymmetric category pair' (see Appendix A). Basically, this means that the two parties to the relationship do not have access to the same knowledge. Here, for example, the author enjoys access to a much greater degree of knowledge than the reader, and thus occupies a position of authority and power. This has the consequence that the author has the capacity to control and organize the reader's encounter with the text and, thus, the power to influence the meaning and interpretation attributed to certain events.

A further feature contributing to the authoritative status of the author, as embodied within the Author's Note, consists of its 'reflective' stance towards past events. This is apparent through use of the *Present* Perfect tense, which serves to capture both an 'enduring present', *un present qui dure*, and a gap between the past and the future. For example, a distinction is drawn between past knowledge and present knowledge, between what the author *knew then* and what the author *knows now*. This distinction is indicated through the repeated use of temporal markers, for example: '*until three years ago*'; '*recently* recovered memories'; 'I *now* understand it'; and '*after all*'. Here we have an *ex post facto* position, a retrospective stance, affording a perspective that was inaccessible to both Fraser and other participants involved in the relevant events *at the time when they were actually occurring*. In this way, Fraser casts herself as an 'observer' of past events – an observer who has the benefit of hindsight and is, therefore, able to look at those events from an 'objective' standpoint.

The Author's Note provides the reader with the impression that there is someone standing behind the statements made within the text; a person lending credence and authority to those statements. Goffman (1981) refers to this impression as the 'textual self'. As will become clear within this chapter, however, this 'textual self' is not confined to the Author's Note, but appears at periodic intervals throughout the text. On each of these occasions, the 'textual self' performs a formulating role, a role which provides a definitive and authoritative version of events. For this reason, I have called this 'textual self' the 'interpretive voice'.

Other Voices

A number of 'other' voices are present in Fraser's account. It is important to note that these 'voices' are all interconnected within the text. Their separation and the treatment of them as individual and independent entities is entirely the product of my analytic orientation towards the account. Any 'competent' reading of the text would require that the voices be read in interaction with each other, as they are, ultimately, inseparable. They gain their meaning and their significance from their relationship to each other. In Bakhtin's terms, they form a 'dialogical relationship' – a 'polyglot world': each of them throws light upon each other; one voice can, after all, see itself only in the light of another voice (Bakhtin, 1981, p. 12). The voices form a system in which they mutually and ideologically interanimate one another.

The voices within Fraser's text, all of which use the first-person pronoun 'I', reflect the influence of a psychoanalytic framework on the text, for the voices can be seen as representative of the tripartite model of the mind set out by Freud. The interpretive voice referred to earlier in relation to the Author's Note, for instance, represents the integrated, balanced ego or psyche (the whole, 'healed', authorial self). Additionally, there are two other voices within the text. The first I have called the 'narrative voice'. This represents the 'persona' – an aspect of the person as shown to or perceived by others (otherwise known as the 'super-ego' – that part of the self which acts as a conscience and responds to externally imposed social rules). The second I have called the 'unconscious voice' and this represents the 'personal unconscious' – that part of the mind which is inaccessible to the conscious mind but which affects behaviour and emotions (otherwise known as the 'id').

The narrative voice uses the present tense and, throughout the text, portrays the protagonist at various stages of chronological development; at each stage of the story the vocabulary and style Fraser deploys are those that would have been available to Sylvia herself at that point in her biographical development (NB: throughout this book I use 'Fraser' to refer to the author herself, and 'Sylvia' when referring to her as a character within *My Father's House*). For instance, in the first chapter which portrays the author's early childhood, this voice begins: 'I sit on my daddy's lap playing ticktacktoe' (p. 3). And then in a later chapter portraying adolescence: 'We walk to Hamilton High, hugging our loose-leaf notebooks to our chest in the female style, thus squelching any rumour that we might have breasts ...' (p. 66). And, as a pretentious student, in the language of philosophers:

> Five other students share my philosophy course, five other talking heads ... we sit in the rec hut over black coffee, and these are the things we say:
> 'Are you implying that Thomas Aquinas is absurd?'
> 'He builds a beautifully coherent system of logic on premises so holey they look like Swiss cheese'.
> 'But if you eliminate God you're left with a solipsism ...'.
> (p. 124)

Thus, the narrative voice portrays an ongoing stream of action – the 'Here and Now' which is still in the making as the text progresses. The characterization of events within this voice is confined to the partial temporal field associated with the relevant biographical stage of development.

The unconscious voice (marked by the use of italics) serves as a means of solving a technical difficulty within the text. It is essential that the reader should have access to the knowledge of sexually abusive events as the narrative progresses, because the impact of such events is crucially dependent upon their temporal placement. How, then, given that the narrative voice and self is ignorant of such events (due to repression and the splitting of personality at around the age of seven), is the reader to be allowed access to such knowledge after this stage of biographical development has passed? The ignorance of the narrative voice must be maintained in order to preserve the narrative voice's 'eyewitness principle' – i.e. a 'negative rule' in which 'the artist must not include in his image anything the eyewitness could not have seen from a particular point at a particular moment' (Gombrich cited in Bann, 1987, pp. 85–6).[3]

The 'unconscious voice' solves this problem. This voice also uses the

present tense, thus maintaining the narrative voice's strategy of documenting events from an ongoing experiential and subjective perspective.
The unconscious voice is repeatedly interpolated into the narrative voice
which gives an impression of spontaneity; of the seepage of knowledge
from unconsciousness into consciousness. For example:

> Now Joe links arms, forcing me to even greater intimacy and an
> even slower beat, *and making my other self very, very nervous.*
> *She cannot bear to be held or confined'.* (p. 44)

> My father calls me into his bedroom. *Since my mother is also in*
> *the house, my other self understands it is me he is calling and not*
> *her.* (p. 95)

In this way the reader gains access to knowledge of sexual events taking
place within childhood and adolescence, knowledge which is denied to
the narrative voice.

It should be clear from this brief introduction to the voices that the
narrative and the unconscious voice and, relatedly, the parts of the self
that they represent (i.e. 'super-ego' and 'id'), coexist in tension in Fraser's
text, continuously producing conflicting testimonies as to 'what really
happened'. Given the existence of such conflict, which version of the
event does the reader accept as representative of the 'true' state of affairs?
Are both versions accepted as equally representative of reality? Or,
alternatively, is one version upheld as representative of the 'truth'?

Earlier in this chapter I referred to the interpretive voice of the
Author's Note, which was characterized as occupying a formulating role
within the text. The interpretive voice, as I have already suggested,
represents the whole of the psyche. This voice opens almost every
chapter, continually characterizing 'what has been talked about so far',
thus making explicit the significance of certain events that have taken
place within foregoing sections of the account. However, the main
characteristic feature of the interpretive voice is the fact that it represents
the 'normal', 'healed', 'repaired' and unitary self; it represents Fraser as
she is now – fully functioning, fully competent and successful. In other
words, this voice represents the central 'world' of the text. As such, the
interpretive voice enjoys access to a whole range of tacit cultural
knowledge as befits any mature, competent member of society. Hence,
within this voice, we encounter knowledge of morally 'appropriate'
standards of behaviour as regards certain 'types' of persons and certain
'kinds' of places; of the 'who', 'where', 'what', 'when', 'why' – the taken-
for-granted knowledge through and by which we make sense of the

social world. It is access to such knowledge that comprises a crucial *starting point* for the interpretive voice's accounting for both ongoing and past behaviour. Crucially, it is from this standpoint that a number of assumptions which govern the whole understanding of events within the text are operative.

One of the most central assumptions is the notion that an inherent, subjective self can be found at the very core of a person's existence. As Kohut puts it:

> [we may recognise] ... the simultaneous existence of contra- dictory selves: of different selves of various degrees of stability and of various degrees of importance. There are conscious, pre- conscious and unconscious selves.... Among these selves, however, there is one which is most centrally located in the psyche; one which is experienced as the basic one, and which is most resistant to change. I like to call this the 'nuclear self'. (Kohut cited in Crews, 1986, p. 33)

In Fraser's text, for instance, as I have already suggested, multiple 'selves' and multiple experiences of reality are encountered. Within the narrative voice, the self of the 'I' is constantly subject to change. There is the 'I' of the child self, the 'I' of the adolescent self, the 'I' of the adult self, etc. Additionally, throughout the text there is the psychological 'other self' of the unconscious voice.

However, despite these varieties of 'self' and the varieties of reality which they represent, it is the 'I' of the interpretive voice that is authoritative throughout the course of *My Father's House.* It is this 'I' which remains constant over the course of the text. It is this 'I', the 'I' of the textual self, that comprises the definitive unity, the null point, the coordinate point in space and time, from which all other 'versions' of reality, from all other 'parts' of the self, are judged. Hence, from the authoritative standpoint of the interpretive voice, the various 'I's' of the narrative voice are seen as 'partial' and 'other'.

This is evident in terms of the fact that the interpretive voice is able to categorize past parts of herself represented in the narrative voice, as an outside observer might do. For example, the interpretive voice refers to past parts of the self as a 'seven-year-old baby' and a 'glamour girl'. This serves as a crucial mechanism by which the interpretive voice can distance herself from the past. In Mead's terms the past actions of the self are grasped, from the standpoint of the present subject 'I', in terms of the 'me'; the 'object' of the past. In the act of reflection, the retrospective turn, the 'self' can only be grasped at an earlier phase of development.

In reflecting on myself, therefore, I can only attend to myself as an object for reflection, and, in doing so, the unity of previous actions and previous 'selves' falls to pieces. In Schutz's terms:

> The self which performed the past acts is no longer the undivided total self, but rather a partial self, the performer of this particular act that refers to a system of correlated acts to which it belongs. This partial self is merely the taker of a role or – to use with all necessary reserve a rather equivocal term which James and Mead have introduced in the literature – a 'Me'. (Schutz, 1962, p. 216)

It is, however, important to stress that an interactive relationship exists between the interpretive voice and the narrative voice. It is only in terms of the interpretive voice's reflective stance that the narrative voice comes to represent 'merely' a 'me'. If the narrative voice were to be taken in isolation from the interpretive voice, the 'I' of the narrative voice would comprise a unitary self. Similarly, the 'I' of the interpretive voice only achieves the status of a 'healed' self, a 'whole' self, a *transcendental* self, in terms of its juxtaposition with the partial and divided selves of the past (and also the divided psychological self – see later in this chapter). It is in this sense that, as Hegel argued, the notion of the Other is indispensable for the construction of the Self and for self-consciousness. It is also apparent here that the relationship between narrative voice and interpretive voice consists, as in the case of the relationship between reader and author, in an asymmetric category pair. By this, I mean that the interpretive voice has access to more knowledge than that of the narrative voice, and therefore the former enjoys a position of power and authority relative to the latter.

Formulations at the Level of Utterance-by-Utterance

So far, the authoritative role of the interpretive voice has been examined solely at the level of 'topic' or 'theme'. The formulating work of the interpretive voice, however, also takes place, as I suggested earlier in this chapter, interrelatedly, at the level of utterance-by-utterance organiz-ation. This involves an issue often analysed by conversation analysts, called turn-taking. Basically, conversation analysts who are interested in this issue look at the way in which conversations are organized in a manner which makes them orderly, coherent and understandable for those engaging within a particular conversation. One of the devices which has been found underlying the organization of conversations is the 'adjacency pair' (Schegloff and Sacks, 1973, pp. 233–65). The 'adjacency pair' characterizes the way in which questions and answers are organized into sequences in conversational interaction. For example, in an adjacency pair such as 'question–answer' – an 'answer' is always conditional upon the 'question' that preceded it. This is known as a relationship of 'conditional relevance':

> By conditional relevance of one item on another we mean; given the first, the second is expectable, upon its occurrence it can be seen to be a second item to the first; upon its non occurrence it can be seen to be officially absent. (Schegloff, 1972, p. 364)

Two utterances standing in a relationship of conditional relevance to one another comprise an *adjacency pair*. Adjacency pairs have three essential features. First, they have a 'two-utterance length' which basically means that there are two statements in each 'adjacency pair' such as a 'question' and an 'answer'. Second, 'adjacency pairs' are 'positioned adjacently', meaning that, for instance, the 'answer' occurs as a 'response' to the 'question'. And, finally, the third feature of adjacency pairs is that different speakers produce each of the utterances (Schegloff and Sacks, 1973, p. 338).

While this sort of analysis has previously been largely restricted to conversation, it can sometimes also be applied to written texts; Fraser's book is a case in point. The interpretive voice and the narrative voice within Fraser's text produce adjacency pairs, conforming to the three features described above. First, in most chapters of the text there is a two-utterance length. Here, I interpret 'utterance' in a very general sense, using it to refer to a general change in the way in which events are framed within the text, or to when the author alters her standpoint with regard to a certain issue (Goffman, 1981, p. 128). Second, there is also adjacent positioning of utterances. Diagram 1 (see Appendix B) shows the format of the whole text in terms of the organizational sequence of these utterances. As can be seen, the pattern typically runs interpretive voice (IV)/narrative voice (NV) ... IV/NV ... IV/NV ... IV/NV.... However, there are exceptions to this typical positioning of the interpretive voice. These exceptions include: anomalies (A), lengthy stretches (LS) and third turns (TT). Their significance will become clear as the study progresses. The third feature of the adjacency pair is that different speakers produce each utterance of the pair. As has already been suggested in my outline of formulation at the level of topic, the interpretive voice and the narrative voice each portray a different 'speaker' in terms of differential biographical (spatial and temporal) positioning.

Having established that the relationship between the interpretive voice and the narrative voice comprise an adjacency pair, it is possible to address the implications of such pairing. In previous studies it has been shown that the turn-taking system bears a direct relation to the way in which knowledge, and access to knowledge, is controlled. For example, analysis of encounters between physicians and patients on the one hand, and examination of witnesses in courtrooms, on the other, reveal evidence of an institutionalized turn-taking system in which the physician, judge and lawyer have privileged access to the 'questioning' type of turn at talk. As a consequence, people occupying these positions experience greater control over the interactional encounter than their counterparts (i.e. the patient or the defendant). This is because, at the close of each sequence of question–answer pairing, control is given back to the person who will start the next sequence. The expert, having rights to control of the questions, is repeatedly the one to regain control. Thus, as long as one is in the position of having exclusive right to the role of questioner then, in part, one has control of the conversation (Sacks, 1989, p. 107).

These observations make clear that the first position of the interpretive voice within Fraser's text enables it to achieve definitional control over the whole of the text. Hence, it is possible to see the way in which the interpretive voice consists of a *formulation* at both the levels of 'topical' and utterance-by-utterance organization within the text.

Formulations and Deletion: The Invisibility of the 'Objective'

The above overview shows how the interpretive voice gains its formulating and authoritative position in relation to the narrative voice owing to its 'superior' temporal and sequential positioning within the text. Earlier in this chapter, however, I also mentioned another voice: the unconscious voice. Is it the case that the interpretive voice also coexists with this voice in an asymmetrical relationship? On first glance this appears to be the case because the unconscious voice, like the narrative voice, makes use of the present tense. It appears, therefore, not to have access to the retrospective knowledge of the interpretive voice. However, this impression is in itself a product of the formulating work of the interpretive voice.

For example, on closer inspection, it becomes clear that the unconscious voice *does* have access to the same authoritative knowledge as the interpretive voice; knowledge that is denied to the narrative voice. This can be shown by looking at the way in which the unconscious voice makes reference to the divided psychological self. For example, the unconscious voice makes repeated reference to *my other self* and uses the third-person pronouns *she* and *her*. This 'other self' is characterized by the interpretive voice at an early stage within the text as the product of repression which results in the psychological division of consciousness and the splitting of personality. However, as has already been shown in relation to the interpretive voice, it is only possible to 'name' past parts of the self when one takes a retrospective standpoint towards them. Accordingly, the unconscious voice can only refer to the existence of an 'other' self with the adoption of a retrospective stance. Quite clearly, then, the unconscious voice has access to the same knowledge as the interpretive voice. This fact is also evident in the unconscious voice's use of flashbacks and flashforwards, which bring home in no uncertain terms its retrospective and all-encompassing knowledge. For example: '*Though I don't yet know it, my maternal grandfather hanged himself, age forty-four, and a maternal aunt soon would*' (p. 146). Thus, despite the unconscious voice's rhetorical use of the present tense, it shares the same retrospective position as the interpretive voice.

This, however, is certainly not the impression of the unconscious voice put forward by the formulating, interpretive voice in the Author's Note. Here, the reader is informed that: 'I have used italics (the unconscious voice) to indicate *thoughts, feelings and experiences* pieced together from recently recovered *memories*, and to indicate *dreams*'. Moreover, the reader is instructed that it is important to keep this device in mind when reading *My Father's House*. Clearly, the message here is that the reader must bear in mind that italicized text represents knowledge deriving from the author's 'inner', private subjectivity; knowledge emerging from the mysterious and elusive sources of the 'id' (represented by the unconscious voice). This impression is further buttressed by Fraser's claim that, as a result of amnesia, much of her story remained unknown to her until three years earlier. As will become clear as my analysis progresses, Fraser's knowledge that she was sexually abused as a child is seen as *deriving*, mysteriously and spontaneously, from 'subjective' sources.

What is significant about the fact that the unconscious voice operates from a retrospective standpoint, whilst giving the impression of spontaneity? The significance of this can be shown by drawing on Coulter's

(1983) analysis of what he calls 'opacity/transparency elisions'.[4] He uses the following example:

> If I were to say of my pre-linguistic infant that he is watching the President on television, it is clear that I am describing the object of his watching from an *adult* point of view, which is one that he cannot literally be said to have ... I am conflating the way it is with the child with the way it is for me (and you) as a socialised concept user. The opaque version of the child's perception may be rendered as 'watching *' where * can have a value only within the domain of concept users (e.g. 'The President'). The transparent version of the child's perceptions (the one true for the observer) is simply that the child is watching the President on television, *only the implication of putting it this way is that is also opaquely true (i.e. true for the child himself)*. (Coulter, 1983, pp. 108–9)

Coulter argues that when an opaque description (one true for the pre-linguistic infant) is substituted by a transparent description (one true for the adult but not necessarily for the pre-linguistic infant), then problems can arise because the 'transparent' description does not necessarily maintain the *truth value* of the pre-linguistic infant's way of seeing things. The related concept of *de re/de dicto* highlights the importance of the question of truth value. *De re* means 'about the thing' and *de dicto* means 'about what is said (about the thing)'. The 'transparent' version described in Coulter's example is the '*de dicto*' version because it is what the adult says about the infant, i.e. that she is watching the president on television. It is, however, treated as the *de re* version (or the 'opaque' version), i.e. what the child actually perceives. Here, it can be seen that the substitution of the *de re* version of events, for the *de dicto* version, may lead to an 'elision' – in other words, a failure to appreciate the way in which the pre-linguistic infant understands the world.

How is this relevant to an understanding of the relationship between the unconscious and the interpretive voice? In Coulter's example, the 'adult' point of view is characterized as the authoritative version of events because of its capacity to formulate, via language, what the pre-verbal child is actually doing. Similarly, as I have already demonstrated, the interpretive voice inhabits a formulating role in terms of its ability to inform the reader about the significance of events occurring within the domain of 'other' voices. In this way, the interpretive voice is analogous to the 'adult' point of view, to the transparent or the *de dicto* version of events. On the other hand, the unconscious voice, which represents the 'id' part of the psyche, is analogous to the pre-linguistic infant, to the opaque, or the *de re* version of events because it represents the 'non-conceptual' and the non-linguistic part of the self (i.e. the unconscious). However, the fact that the unconscious voice is infiltrated by the retrospective knowledge of the interpretive voice means that it is the 'adult' or the 'objective' viewpoint which is used to portray 'subjective' or unconscious experience. In other words, the 'opaque' version of events is substituted for by the 'transparent' version of events. The important point to note here is that the version of events provided by the interpretive voice may be incomplete because it fails to take account of the child's 'original' experience and understanding of events.

Moreover, because the unconscious voice is presented *as though* it were a 'direct' and spontaneous expression of events occurring within the author's 'personal subjectivity' (in the Author's Note we are told that italics are used to 'indicate thoughts, feelings and experiences'), this problem is further prevented from coming to light. It is simply assumed that the unconscious voice represents a direct expression of the reality of events which occurred in the past. This assumption means that not only may certain aspects of that reality be omitted from consideration, but also that the reader will fail to notice such omissions and, perhaps, the possible reasons for them.

As is apparent in the Author's Note, Fraser is concerned to emphasize the fact that the 'truth' of her autobiography derives from 'personal experience' and 'subjective knowledge'; the 'truth' emerges from thoughts, feelings and dreams. Accordingly, Fraser shies away from depicting her version of events as a 'full or balanced characterisation'. Rather, her stated aim is '*only* to portray such persons and myself as our lives relate to this difficult story'. Having made such claims, however, Fraser is then concerned to emphasize the fact that her account *does* represent the truth. She tells us that she has not 'exaggerated', 'distorted' or 'misrepresented' the truth as she now understands it. In order to substantiate her claim to truth Fraser refers to independent witnesses. For example, she tells us that the fact that she was sexually abused by her father has now been corroborated by 'outside sources'.

The important point to note here, however, is the way in which the 'subjective', the *de re*, is continually distanced from the 'objective', the *de dicto*. The impression given by Fraser's account is that objective corroboration appears *only after* the truth has emerged from her 'subjective' and 'personal' memories. This can be further demonstrated with reference to a recent review which reports an interview with Fraser and points towards some problems encountered by her in the writing of the memoir. Mackay states that:

Even after she realised she had to write an autobiography, her approach relied too heavily on the critical and distanced eye of her older, wiser consciousness. It became obvious that she was trying to write two books at the same time – an analytic one and an emotional one. (Mackay, 1987, p. 3)

Fraser is then reported as saying that she decided to go for the personal book (Mackay, 1987, p. 3). Here we can see Fraser upholding a distinction between the 'personal' (subjective) and the 'analytic' (objective) versions of events. Moreover, she claims that the authority of *My Father's House* derives from the former. Mackay proceeds to uphold this distinction, suggesting that Fraser's decision to write a personal book, untainted by analysis:

... was a good choice. Her *adult analysis* (interpretive voice) is infrequent, most often a paragraph or two at the opening of the chapter, and it doesn't overwhelm the tone of the book: The analytic passages are *insightful* and *honest*, offering keen perceptions about the less obvious effects of her experience on her and her entire family. (1987, p. 3)

Here, it is clear that the reviewer equates 'adult analysis' with the interpretive voice appearing at the beginning of each chapter. The reviewer fails to recognize the fact that the unconscious voice (which appears throughout the text at crucial points), also consists of 'adult analysis' as opposed to 'pure' emotional outpourings as the text leads one to believe.

The crucial question to ask at this point is why is this separation between the 'personal' and the 'analytic', between the 'subjective' and the 'objective', so important? What exactly does Fraser achieve in her maintenance of this separation? By casting herself into an authoritative role, Fraser commits herself both to the assets, for instance, the capacity to make claims to truth, but also to the liabilities associated with such knowledge, for instance, accountability and responsibility. This means that Fraser must constantly monitor the practical and moral implications that her claims to knowledge might have.[5] For instance, one of the characteristic ways in which people discredit other people's accounts or versions of events is by asking the question 'Who benefits?'. In order to answer this question it would be necessary to 'locate' or 'ground' both the speaker, and the speaker's version of events, within a specific context – in order to ascertain the meaning and significance of the claim. In the light of this possibility, therefore, Fraser is concerned not only to produce an authoritative version of events, but also to account for the grounding of her authority. The introduction of the unconscious voice within the text serves as a means whereby knowledge claims can be simultaneously located and dislocated. This is because knowledge is located within the domain of Fraser's 'private', 'inner' and 'natural' source – the unconscious. At the same time, this means that knowledge is dislocated from the public domain. Hence, knowledge is attached to the individual's psychology and detached from the situation (Smith, 1974). This adds not only to the veracity of the account[6] but also has practical consequences in terms of the ability to question and challenge the author's claims to knowledge. If the grounds on which a truth claim is based are made available to other people, then the claim can be challenged and defended by reference to commonly shared principles. However, in the absence of such information, the possibility of challenge and public debate is considerably reduced. It is on this basis that experiential knowledge claims can be described as 'irresponsible'.

As this chapter has shown, however, it is possible to render 'responsible' such knowledge claims by locating some of the linguistic resources on which they are based. In this way, it becomes clear that just as the astronomers' 'discovery' of the pulsar at the Steward Observatory Laboratory (see Chapter 1), was shown to be tied to certain practices and procedures, so too is Fraser's 'own', 'personal' truth and the 'discovery' of that truth. However, these practices only become apparent through a detailed analysis of Fraser's text because they are consistently 'dis-attended', 'lost' or 'forgotten' over the course of the account.

Conclusion

In this chapter I have examined the way in which authority is established within the text of *My Father's House*. I have shown that this is achieved through the patterning of different voices within the text. Furthermore, I have demonstrated that the sequencing and temporal perspective of the interpretive voice is critical for its authoritative position in relation to the other voices. Simultaneously, however, I have also emphasized the fact that the grounds on which the interpretive voice's authority is based are not made accessible to the reader. This is because Fraser is concerned that her 'truth' should be seen as pre-existent, essential and 'natural'. In the chapters that follow I will be concerned to show how this conception of truth affects the text's thematic development.

Notes

1. A memoir is defined as 'a historical account written from *personal knowledge* or *special sources*' (*OED*, 1991).
2. Lejeune has described this 'entente' between reader and writer as an 'autobiographical pact' (cited in Eakin, 1985, p. 20). He suggests that this 'contract' determines our manner of reading the text, creating the effects that, attributed to the text, seem to define it as autobiography. Lejeune's view has been confirmed by Holland whose experiments showed that reader responses vary 'according to the expectation or "set" the reader brings (to a given text) . . . one kind of "set" for non-fiction, another for fiction' (cited in Eakin, 1985, p. 20). As Graham Watson argues, facticity is a status rather than a self-evident condition. The distinction between fact and fiction is constituted by means embedded in our texts, such as forewords, footnotes and other subtle rhetorical devices which proclaim them as works of non-fiction, and also by means of interpretive practices that readers bring to bear on these instructions (Watson, 1987, p. 458). Similarly, Wittgenstein observed:

    > The criteria for the truth of the *confession* that I thought such-and-such are not criteria for a true *description* of a process. And the importance of the true confession does not reside in its being a correct and certain report of a process. It resides rather in the special consequences which can be drawn from a confession whose truth is guaranteed by the special criteria of *truthfulness* (Wittgenstein, 1953, p. 222).

3. Bakhtin refers to such techniques as 'plot interest' (the condition of not knowing) in relation to the novel. He suggests that the novel devises various forms and methods for employing the surplus knowledge that the author has, that which the hero or the protagonist does not know or does not see (Bakhtin, 1981, p. 32).
4. The terms 'opacity' and 'transparency' are taken from W.V. Quine (1960). The 'elision' arises when an opaque version of something (i.e. a version true for the perceiver) is conflated with a transparent version (i.e. a version true for the observer of the perceiver) (cited in Jalbert, 1982, p. 165).
5. In Garfinkel's terms, we are allowed 'no time out' (Garfinkel, 1967). And, in Sacks's terms: 'members of society are constantly engaged in monitoring events; on the one hand by reference to whether something that has happened is something they're accountable for, and on the other hand, to find out what is getting done by members of any of the other categories' (Sacks, 1989, p. 273).
6. This finding contrasts with a recent review written by Hak on the book *At the Will of the Body: Reflections on Illness* by Frank. Hak suggests that the impact of the book will be reduced because Frank argues mainly from his illness experience and not by referring to arguments and evidence within the sociological and philosophical literature (Frank is a medical sociologist). According to Hak: 'Frank risks the danger that his opinions will be read as merely the personal view of a patient who has discovered the value of life and illness by experiencing cancer' (Hak, 1992, p. 18). My analysis shows, by contrast, that an appeal to personal experience can serve to increase the veracity and impact of the book rather than to diminish it. I am not arguing that the same holds in relation to Frank's account, but it is important to recognize that the appeal to personal experience can be used as an authorizing strategy in its own right.

Chapter 4

Step One: The 'Public' Location of the Problem

Introduction

In Chapter 2 I highlighted the fact that Fraser's text is premised upon the three-step model of psychoanalytic procedure *Recollection, Repetition and Working Through*. In this chapter, attention is focused upon the first section of the text which represents the first step of that procedure, namely *Recollection*. This selection of the text could be described as the 'primary narrative' because it provides the framework and the essential background details on which later sections of the text will 'work'.

In Chapter 2 I also pointed out that one reviewer of Fraser's text had interpreted it as representative of the socialist feminist position with regard to issues of childhood sexual abuse. In this chapter, I look at the way in which Fraser's text could be interpreted in this way. However, I then argue that such an interpretation fails to take account of the *formal* organization of the text, by which I mean the organization of various 'voices' within the text (see Chapter 3). The organization of various voices is highly important because it has a significant impact on the way in which the issue of childhood sexual abuse is interpreted and presented to the reader. As will become clear in this chapter, the authoritative interpretive voice (the voice representing the author's contemporary perspective) plays a major role in this interpretive process. Moreover, in this chapter, we see that the interpretation put forward by this 'voice' is related to a wider historical 'discourse'. On this basis, I argue that not only does the failure to take account of the textual organization of voices result in a misinterpretation of Fraser's text, but it also fails to take account of historical changes leading to differing interpretations of the nature of childhood sexual abuse.

The Personal is Political

Is there any evidence to support the idea that Fraser's text represents a socialist feminist perspective regarding the issue of childhood sexual abuse? In the last chapter I showed how, within Fraser's text, there are a number of voices, each representing a different version of reality. One of these voices was the narrative voice. To recap, this voice changes its nature over the course of *My Father's House*. This is because, as its name suggests, the narrative voice 'narrates' the course of events from an experiential or 'subjective' viewpoint. This viewpoint changes in accordance with the biographical stage of life that is being represented at any particular point within the text. Thus, for example, the narrative voice portrays experiences of events as they are experienced by Sylvia Fraser as a child, an adolescent, a student, a young married woman, a divorced woman, etc. At each stage within the text, the narrative voice attempts to portray events as they would have been experienced by Sylvia Fraser at the time when they were actually occurring.

It is in relation to the version of events provided by the narrative voice in the first section of the text that *My Father's House* can be interpreted as representative of the socialist feminist discourse. However, it is important to emphasize that such an interpretation is based *only* on the narrative voice's portrayal within this selected portion of the text. I now proceed to examine this in more detail.

As I suggested in the last chapter, the narrative voice portrays certain 'personae' over the course of the text. The first 'persona' is of Sylvia Fraser as a child. Here, it is clear that the portrayal of the experiential or personal 'world' of childhood is solidly located within the 'public' context of the patriarchal nuclear family. Both Sylvia and her mother are characterized as subordinates with regard to the authority of the father. For example: 'My father sits in his fetch-me chair. . . . He grunts: "Fetch me a paring knife". . . . My father sharpens his pencil. "Take this back".' (p. 13). The mother is mainly portrayed as a subservient housewife, dependent upon her husband for his economic support. This is made explicit in a scene when the child rebels against her father's sexual demands:

> *Desperation makes be bold. At last I say the won't-love-me words: 'I'm going to tell my mommy on you!' My father replaces bribes with threats: 'If you do, you'll have to give me back all your toys.' I tot up my losses: my Blondie and Dagwood cutouts, my fairytale colouring book, my crayons.*
> *'My mommy gave those things to me. They're mine.'*

'I paid for them. Everything in this house belongs to me. . . . Your mother will do what I say. . . .' (p. 11)

As one reads about the experiences suffered by the young child at the hands of her father, one is made increasingly aware of the child's growing sense of panic, fear and helplessness as she is locked further within her father's power. For example, near the beginning of the chapter the reader hears the innocent voice of the child as she tells us that: 'My daddy squeezes my legs between his knees. I count my pennies, already imagining them to be blackballs and liquorice from the Candy Factory. . . . *My daddy and I share secrets*' (p. 6). As the chapter progresses, however, so too does the child's heightening sense of fear and frustration: '*His sweat drips on me. I don't like his wet-ums. His wet-ums splashes me . . . I'm afraid to complain because daddy won't love me won't love me won't love me*' (p. 11). And:

> *Now when daddy plays with me I keep my eyes tightly scrunched so I can't see. I don't want his pennies or his candies or his cookies. Mostly I leave them by the pillow while he swallows me. I hold my breath to keep me from crying because daddy won't love me love me love me.* (p. 11)

It is in relation to scenes such as the above that the child is clearly portrayed in a manner which emphasizes her subordinate position relative to the powerful position occupied by the father as head of the family, i.e. as patriarch.

Moreover, as Sylvia gets older and begins to attend school, it becomes evident that the sexual abuse perpetrated upon her by her father is not simply an anomalous event; it is not simply an idiosyncratic feature of her own 'deviant' father or her own 'dysfunctional' family. At school she comes into contact with another sexually abused child, Magda Lunt, who is classed as a reject by the other children: '"Magda's father beats her up. Phew! Magda stinks of fish."' (p. 20). Sylvia stands on the sidewalk: 'Magda doesn't stink of fish. I know that smell. I've smelled it on myself. It's the stink of . . . *fear.* It's the stink of . . . *daddy won't love me love me . . .*' (p. 20). And later that day when Sylvia looks at her 'bright-penny public self' in the mirror:

> A spot clouds the mirror. I rub. It grows larger. I scrub harder. Now I see a smudge where my face used to be. For an instant it turns into a girl who looks like Magda, with thumbprint bruises and fangs for teeth. When I try to rub her out, she lays her warty

palm against mine: 'I'm your partner! I'm your partner!'. (p. 20)

The two young girls are locked in partnership by virtue of the abusive events perpetrated upon them by their fathers. The experience of childhood sexual abuse is not simply a 'private' experience; rather, by contrast, the narrative implies a growing awareness of the fact that such 'private' experiences may represent a more collective phenomenon. This interpretation of events is further buttressed by the fact that Sylvia is not only sexually abused by her father, but also by Mr Brown, a lodger who stays in her father's house during the summer of 1944.

This emphasis on the collectivity of girls' and women's experiences – an emphasis characteristic of the socialist feminist discourse, continues throughout the portrayal of the early and later adolescent years. In fact, it should be emphasized that it is over the course of these years that the portrayal of events from the perspective of socialist feminism reaches its peak. This is expressed in the form of a critique of the hypocrisy of the moral values of the 1950s which revolved around the 'cult of the virgin' and the moral distinction drawn between 'good' girls and 'bad' girls; between the 'virgin' and the 'whore'. By highlighting the hypocrisy of these moral values, Fraser is concerned to tie the abusive experiences suffered by girls and women into the historical and cultural context of patriarchy; the 'personal' is portrayed as a thoroughly 'political' affair.

As I have suggested previously, this is a particularly prevalent theme in the portrayal of the adolescent years. Here, the reader encounters a world dominated by male power. Such power is thematized in terms of male violence, male ownership and possession. For example, Sylvia's experience of adolescence is totally dominated by boys and men engaging in sexually insulting behaviour. She is sexually assaulted by two boys in the cinema as hands 'claw' at her sweater and 'dive' under her skirt (p. 50). Sylvia is also verbally assaulted as one boy tells her: '"Next time you better be wearing tin pants because we're going to work you over so good you'll ..."' (p. 57). Sexually abusive language is also directed towards Sylvia and other cheerleaders as they support their school football team. As they cheerlead at the side of the football pitch, obscenities 'unroll like used toilet paper':

'That's right, Blondie. Get those tits moving!'
The crowd gives a nervous guffaw. Other voices chime in:
'Crotch! Crotch! Give us CROTCH.' (p. 88)

As cheerleaders, Sylvia describes the girls as having a 'a self mocking awareness of the colossal hypocrisy of which we are the eager butts'

(p. 70). Another incident of sexual harassment takes place in a street-car: 'A face presses up to mine, insolent and confident: 'Oh, this one's hot for it. She's really loving it, aren't you, baby?' (p. 99). Further incidents of sexual harassment are evident. For example, a defaced school election poster upon which, 'My lips have been reddened, my hair painted gold. The caption, EXPERIENCE COUNTS, has been altered to read EXPERI-ENCED CUNT' (p. 91). Sylvia also receives dirty phone-calls and poison-pen letters. Indeed, it is in relation to such widespread practices of objectification that the narrative is able to draw an analogy between the father's abusive acts against Sylvia and those which exist in society at large. For example, when Sylvia's father first attempts full penetrative intercourse, Sylvia is described as feeling:

> ... *used, not as one person exploited by another, but as a condom is used then discarded in the gutter ... She is old enough, now, to understand how completely she has been betrayed.* (p. 43)

Connections are also drawn between economics, sex, possession and freedom. For example, waiting to go into the cinema Sylvia remembers 'the first rule of dating: loss of economic freedom equals loss of personal freedom' (pp. 48–9). At a raided pyjama party, boys huddle along the wall looking on while the girls are 'Humiliated at having to hang around like merchandise when nobody is buying' (p. 61). At the Fall Frolic, boys buy the girls corsages:

> Like all the other girls I know the code: orchids at $4.00 to $6.50 for show-offs; gardenias, like mine, at $3.50 for sophisticates; roses at $3.00 for going-steady couples; $2.50 for casual dates; no corsage – a confession of poverty and/or no manners, an insult. (p. 81)

At the school dance Sylvia feels as if she is 'possessed' by her date as his arms 'coil possessively' around her, constricting her like 'clamps'. And when she dances with someone other than her date, we are informed that this is not usual practice because the 'financial investment' is so high at the school dance. After having being 'returned' to her date, she feels guilty '*like Daddy's naughty girl who's failed to please*' (p. 86). Moreover, Sylvia feels an obligation to 'give her services' to her date as he takes her home after the school dance:

> This shouldn't be first-date stuff, but I've been adding up the
> gasoline and the corsage ... and I find something owing which,
> being an honest tradeswoman, I feel obliged to deliver. (p. 86)

Continuing this theme of male possession and ownership, the father is
portrayed as having ownership of his family. Accordingly, Sylvia, her
mother and her sister are expected to service him. The father sits in his
armchair 'as if it were his throne', ordering his wife and daughters to
fetch things for him – well-iced King Cola, the paper, his glasses. Fraser
parodies the situation by seeing it as analogous to that in the nursery
rhyme, 'Old King Cole and his Fiddlers Three' (p. 77). Male possession
and domination are thus related, in this part of the text at least, to
economic power.[1]

Ideological power, the power to determine language, thought and
reality, is also portrayed as inextricably bound up with such economic
power. Hence, from this perspective, men have the power to determine
reality. This reality is the reality encountered by Sylvia's adolescent self,
which the narrative calls 'Appearances'. 'Appearances' is geared towards
the satisfaction of male-defined standards. Sylvia and other girls see
themselves and others through the 'male gaze' (p. 64). Because 'Holly-
wood agrees' that gentlemen prefer blonde hair, for Appearances,
blonde hair is 'standard equipment' (p. 75). Because dating is the
standard by which Sylvia's high school, Hamilton High, judges a girl's
popularity, Appearances fills her date book 'like a junkie' (p. 65). Sylvia's
friend, Babs, goes on a diet in order to model herself into 'something the
boys don't mind being seen with'. Consequently, she fails her exams and
her conversation is reduced to talking about dates and calories.

Over this part of the text, a resounding theme is that the reality
experienced by each girl or woman in a male-dominated world takes on
an increasing form of artificiality or non-reality. Sylvia is characterized·as
feeling weary owing to the constant pressures of presentation required
by Appearances; she feels as if she is continually preparing for a part in
a play. Similarly, her friend, Lulu, is characterized as 'always playing a
part. Like me' (p. 81). Sylvia and her friends are all institutionalized into
the male-dominated version of reality. Accordingly, they are characterized as ephemeral 'talking heads' with no substance. As they enter
Hamilton High for their final six months, they can be found 'talking,
talking, talking' but 'saying nothing'.

As is to be expected with people who feel they have no stake or
share in the dominant version of reality, such experiences result in a
mixture of confused rage, anger, guilt and fear. Rage 'pours out' of Sylvia,
'like lava, devastating everything in its path' (p. 46). Her rage builds and

is fuelled by its 'underground source' (p. 57). The adolescent Sylvia tells the reader that she hates her father. Her hate derives from her unconscious 'other self' and this is made clear through the use of the unconscious voice (italicized text): '*I hate you father.* Let me count the ways . . .' (p. 77). The text becomes increasingly disjointed and fragmentary as the boundaries between appearance and reality break down and the threat of craziness and mental breakdown looms overhead: 'Now the split between what I am and what I pretend to be is so wide I can barely straddle the gap' (p. 101).

Anger and frustration are expressed in the form of self-harm as the adolescent Sylvia claims that she can burn her arm with a cigarette and not feel anything. She can wrap her arm around pain 'till it smothers in its own scream'. One of these days, she tells us, she will 'blot out this whole fucking universe' (p. 101). Sylvia also ceases to menstruate. She is reduced to 98 pounds. It is important here, however, to stress the fact that the hysteria suffered by Sylvia is not an experience suffered solely by her. Rather, such experience constitutes more of a 'collective' experience. Sylvia's friends are characterized as suffering in a similar manner. They too are victims of the patriarchal system. Babs is suffering from anorexia and bad nerves and Lulu is pregnant but trying desperately to deny it. She has worn the same box-pleated skirt and blazer for a month, attempting to hold her books against her stomach to hide the bulge. Meanwhile she continues to rehearse for the school play *Romeo and Juliet* in which she is playing the lead part, Juliet. As is apparent in the following quote, here, the text creates a heightening sense of fragmentation, hysteria and collective madness.

> Sometimes Lulu swoons so deeply Boris Wayne and Herb Swamp practically have to revive her. Then she looks up at me and winks – or does she? She knows I'm there – or does she? And I know she knows – or do I? I know she's pregnant – isn't she? And she knows I know – doesn't she? But why does she keep rehearsing? . . . . (p. 100)

The culminating point of the rage and hatred experienced by Sylvia as an adolescent is expressed in a scene where Sylvia is forced by her father to perform oral sex. In the course of this encounter, Sylvia is characterized as being overcome by a total sense of rage as her 'other self' takes over consciousness. This is clear in the following quote from this scene in which the unconscious voice claims that the rage experienced by the 'other self' is:

> *Not rage projected against her mother or the teachers or the boys
> at Hamilton High or herself, which is the kind of rage I always
> feel. No, her rage is directed at the person who caused that rage,
> who still causes it. . . . As daddy pushes her head down to his
> crotch, she at last gets out the words: 'I hate you!' . . . . (p. 103)*

It is of the utmost importance here to note where Sylvia's rage and anger
is directed. It is directed at her father. It is directed against the person
who has perpetrated sexual abuse upon her for over 10 years. Sylvia
holds him, and only him, responsible for his actions. This, I suggest, is
to some extent the result of adopting a socialist feminist perspective
towards the events experienced by women and girls in the context of a
male-dominated and patriarchal society. It is important to bear this point
in mind because it will become increasingly significant at later stages in
the analysis.

For the time being, however, I will move on to complete my survey
of the extent to which the first section of Fraser's text can be said to
provide a socialist feminist perspective on the issue of childhood sexual
abuse. As has just become clear, the adolescent years are portrayed as a
mixture of fear and frustration deriving from male social, economic and
ideological power. This fear eventually results in hysteria, and almost
leads to Sylvia's total mental breakdown. Just as this is about to happen,
however, Sylvia meets Danny, her future husband, and she falls in love.
Danny, her 'prince', 'saves' and 'heals' her, leading her away from mental
breakdown. He leads her away from total confusion; away from her
confusion between 'Appearance' and 'Reality'. Indeed, the text suggests
that 'love' has the power to bring forth the real truth, the real 'Reality' of
the world. Love has the power to 'heal'. I will return to this episode in
more detail later. For the moment, however, it is necessary to address the
question of how such 'romantic' imagery connects with the socialist
feminist perspective evident within the text so far. On this point, it is
important to note that the narrative self-effacingly undercuts the suggestion of romance within the text. For example:

> And so the handsome prince kissed the sleeping princess and . . .
> and. . . . No, it doesn't quite work that way. *This is real life after
> all.* (p. 113)

By contrast with such romantic imagery, the text then proceeds to
document the nature of women's 'real-life' experiences of 'love'. In
accordance with the socialist feminist dictate that the 'personal is political',
the narrative ties the 'private' experience of 'love' into the public context.

As Sylvia leaves school and takes on a part-time job in her vacation prior to entering university she learns a 'new vocabulary' – a vocabulary of '*failed rescue*' and of 'unmet hopes' (p. 112). For example, single women yearn for the 'Right Man' to rescue them. They fail to notice that the married women remain 'unrescued'. The married women dream of buying the 'Right House', so that they can rescue their marriages and their children. When one woman goes to church to confess her sins, she tells the priest that she has used a diaphragm. 'You know that's a mortal sin' (p. 112), the priest responds. The woman answers, yes, she knows this, but she had to commit the sin because the last time she became pregnant, her husband beat her up. And finally, in a scene where Sylvia and Danny are alone in his father's house, kissing, Danny tries to persuade Sylvia to make love. But Sylvia does not want to. Consequently, Danny is disappointed and disapproving. In a 'punitive' voice he asks: 'You'd make love if I wanted to, wouldn't you?' (p. 117). Although Sylvia is characterized as feeling 'resentful' and 'manipulated', she forces out the word 'yes'. 'It's a small price to pay for paradise isn't it?' (p. 117), she asks rhetorically. This, then, is the 'reality' of the 'love' encountered by women and girls in the course of their everyday lives. Thus, it appears to be the case that the theme of 'love as reality', or of 'love' having the capacity to 'heal', is undermined as the narrative voice ties 'private' experiences of 'love' into the 'reality' of their 'public', patriarchal context.

The emphasis on the 'public' historical contextualization of events and experiences is maintained as Sylvia's experiences at university are portrayed. The 'cult of the virgin' still lies heavily upon female under-graduates and, 'as always' sex has to do with "them", their needs and our reactions' (p. 129). Their needs and our reactions are, once more, linked to 'their' economic status. The faculties of medicine and business administra-tion ('its undergrads are often scions being groomed to inherit the family empire') are viewed as 'hunting grounds for male selection' because a 'good catch' must include 'guaranteed upper-middle-class income' (p. 122). By contrast, most girls take arts subjects and secretarial science courses which reflect the belief that 'a girl's happiest role is as wife and mother' (p. 121). This belief is espoused by Professor Wynn from the philosophy department, when Sylvia has a discussion with him about career choices. He tells her that she has been living in a 'fool's paradise'. No one, he tells her, takes a woman scholar seriously, especially not in philosophy. Luckily, he comments, Sylvia is engaged. Professor Wynn has always told his wife that the 'simple example' of her sitting before their children reading scholarly material in the original Latin is a better advertisement for a classical education than all of his preaching (p. 136).

From the above overview, then, it is apparent that over the course of the first section of *My Father's House* there is considerable evidence to suggest that Fraser's interpretation of her experience of childhood sexual abuse relies on a socialist feminist perspective. 'Private' experiences are located within their social, historical and economic context. This is evident not only in terms of the themes that I have just outlined, but also in terms of the types of descriptions of people, places and time periods prevalent within the first section of the text. For example, Sylvia's 'personal' development is charted mainly through the use of 'public' chronological benchmarks or biographical stages of development such as 'childhood', 'adolescence', 'student', etc. These stages of develop-ment, in turn, take place in 'public' places such as 'school', 'university' and the 'workplace'. In the first section of the narrative such 'times' and 'places' are mainly described in 'public' or 'official' terms. By this, I mean that the timing of events is specified in terms of dates; for example, at the beginning of the text, as Fraser prepares the reader for her forthcoming 'testimony', she identifies her date of birth: 'I was born into my father's house before noon on March 8, 1935 . . .' (p. 3). Similarly, events occurring during the adolescent years are historically located via specification of the temporal period; for example, 'Fall Frolic '52' and '. . . the pristine and unforgiving fifties' (p. 94). Events are also 'officially' located with regard to the identification of places. This is evident, for example, when proper nouns are used to identify a specific place. For example, Fraser identifies the name of the country and district in which she was born (Hamilton, Ontario), the names of her schools (Laura Secord Public School, Hamilton High), and of the university she attended (University of Western Ontario). The significance of using such 'official' or 'public' descriptions in order to characterize the who, when and where of events will become increasingly apparent as my analysis proceeds. As will become clear, it is the 'public' location of persons, places and times that significantly affects the way in which the experience of childhood sexual abuse is interpreted and, indeed, of the way in which its incidence is accounted for. The significance of the 'public' location of experiential events within Fraser's text, however, only becomes apparent when one considers an alternative character-ization of events evident within *My Father's House*. It is this contrasting characterization of events that I now proceed to outline.

An Alternative Interpretation of Events

So far, then, from the outline I have provided of some of the major themes and issues emerging from *My Father's House*, it does seem as if the interpretation of sexually abusive events is premised upon a socialist feminist perspective. It does seem as if the 'personal' is located within the domain of the 'political'. However, at the beginning of this chapter, I suggested that such an interpretation of Fraser's text fails to take account of the *formal* organization of the text, i.e. of the organization of various 'voices' within the text. When such organizational properties are taken into account, I suggest that the alternative characterization of experiences of childhood sexual abuse alluded to above becomes increasingly apparent.

In Chapter 3, I showed how the interpretive voice occupies a dominant and authoritative role within the text. This authority is manifested in the text in terms of the interpretive voice's ability to formulate the significance of certain events and experiences that have been previously reported by the narrative voice. Given the existence of such authority, it is obvious that an interpretation of Fraser's text which takes account only of experiences and events portrayed within the narrative voice (as just provided above), is woefully inadequate, in that it takes no account of some of the major organizational features of the text. As I will now proceed to demonstrate, when one takes these features into account the whole interpretation of the nature of childhood sexual abuse changes significantly. Moreover, I suggest that the different interpretation of events put forward by narrative voice and the interpretive voice embeds a wider historical shift from a socialist feminist perspective, towards the more contemporary 'healing' discourse. The impact of such a shift will become clear as the analysis proceeds.

Separating 'Public' and 'Private' Reality

In my outline of the first section of the narrative in *My Father's House*, I have suggested that there is an attempt to show the way in which Sylvia's 'private' experience is interconnected with the 'public' socio-historical context. From this perspective, there is no 'inner', 'private' experience that separates or divorces Sylvia Fraser from the experiences of other women and girls living within the same 'public' climate of patriarchy. However, if one takes into consideration the formulations provided by the interpretive voice with regard to the 'public' location of such 'private' experiences, a rather different picture begins to emerge.

This becomes most evident during the adolescent years when the interpretive voice introduces the 'persona' known as 'Appearances'. Rather than conceiving of this 'persona' or social role as essentially connected to the way in which girls and women experience reality (as did the narrative voice), the interpretive voice implies a subtly different interpretation. What begins to emerge is an image of the 'Appearances' persona as *merely* a persona. When a 'social role' or a 'persona' is characterized in this way, the implication is that there is some 'under-lying' private reality separate from the 'public' form of reality embedded within the social world. Indeed, it seems that the interpretive voice is concerned to build up this impression because the 'Appearances' self is described as an *alter ego*. What does this mean – an *alter* ego? An *other* self? I will return to this issue in more detail later. For the time being, however it is important to note that reference to an 'alter ego' assumes the existence of some original, pre-existent 'ego'. Without such an assumption, the notion of an 'alter ego' would make no sense at all. What would the 'alter' be 'alter' to?

It seems, therefore, that the interpretive voice is concerned to draw a distinction between the 'public' part of the self, namely 'Appearances', and another, more 'private' part of the self. This becomes increasingly apparent when the interpretive voice refers to the 'Appearances' self in the third person, using pronouns such as 'she' and 'her', as opposed to the first-person form that is used within the rest of the text. Use of the third person serves an important 'distancing' function, in that it allows Fraser to draw a distinction between the activities performed by 'herself' on the one hand, and those performed by her 'other self', on the other. I will return to such functions at a later stage in the analysis. For the moment, however, it is sufficient to highlight the fact that the interpretive voice is presenting an image, contrary to that presented in some parts of the narrative, of a separation between 'public' and 'private' reality.

In turn, this separation between 'private' and 'public' reality actually feeds into the narrative portrayal of events. This can be demonstrated by reference to a scene taking place between Sylvia and Danny (her future husband). This scene occurs during the midst of Sylvia's increasing sense of dissolving and fragmenting reality described earlier in this chapter. Danny confronts Sylvia asking her if she is in any kind of trouble. He tells her that she is a terrific person and that any guy would be pleased to go out with her. Because of this, he tells her:

> 'You don't have . . . I mean, you've got so much going for you that you don't have to . . . you shouldn't . . .'
> 'Don't have to what?'
> '. . . don't have to . . .'
> 'Say it!'
> '. . . put out for the guys.'
> So here it is at last, the anonymous accusation translated into words.

Filthy, stinking, rotten letters, always anonymous, and even worse phone calls. Oh, this one's hot for it. She's really loving it, aren't you, baby? Repent, repent! The time of Judgment is at hand … That's right Blondie. Get those tits moving! Crotch! Crotch! Give us crotch! WE'RE COMING TO GET YOU SLUT!
I shout: 'It's not true! They're liars!'. (p. 105)

This scene highlights the fact that the image of reality provided by 'Appearances' is not the true version of reality. There is something more to Sylvia behind the appearance. She is not a 'slag', a 'whore', a 'slut', as her adolescent appearance might suggest.

Indeed, it is important to note that Danny believes Sylvia when she tells him that the rumours are not true. This is particularly significant because Danny's belief in the truth of her statement could have a significant impact upon the reader. This is because, throughout the narrative, the character of Danny is built up as representative of the theme of Reality – in contrast to the artificiality of Sylvia's Appearances self. This effect is achieved through a considerable amount of euphemism and idealization in the construction of Danny's character. For example, in the school dance scene, Danny's honesty and genuine character are displayed in contrast with Sylvia's 'play-acting'. Danny admits that he does not like football, being punched or punching people. Sylvia comes to the conclusion that she has nothing to be afraid of: 'Daniel is fun as well as nice. Not a show off like other boys' (p. 83). Euphemistic devices are also employed in the portrayal of Daniel's family, as is clear when Daniel tells Sylvia that his father is a 'wonderful person'. He recalls going on calls with his father (who is a doctor). If it was a poor family, they always took clothes, and every Christmas Danny's father made doll's houses for 'the babies he brought into the world' (p. 110).

Thus, by constructing an image of Danny as a figure whose response the reader can trust, as a figure representing the real state of affairs, the narrative has recourse to a useful persuasive device. When Danny is convinced of the truth of Sylvia's statement, it is more likely that the reader will also be convinced. The important point to note here, however, is the very fact that the narrative is attempting to draw a distinction between the outward 'public' behaviour of Appearances on the one hand, and the 'private' reality of Sylvia's experience on the other. This is a long way from the socialist feminist perspective which attempts to locate such 'private' experiences within the domain of the 'public' social and historical context.

A Distinct 'Private' Reality?

From the above comments it can be seen that when one takes account of the way in which the interpretive voice formulates the nature of the 'Appearances' part of the self, the idea that there is no distinction between 'public' reality and 'private' experience in *My Father's House* cannot be upheld. So far, however, I have refrained from considering the most damning evidence within the text which suggests that such an interpretation is illegitimate. It is this evidence that I shall now turn to.

In the very first chapter of *My Father's House*, both the narrative voice and the unconscious voice inform the reader about some of the traumatic experiences perpetrated upon the child by her father. At the opening of the second chapter, the interpretive voice formulates the impact that those experiences had upon the child in the following manner: 'When the conflict caused by my sexual relationship with my father became too acute to bear, I created a secret accomplice for my daddy by splitting my personality into two' (p. 15). From this point onwards, Sylvia is characterized as living in two separate (and often conflicting) realities. Her 'public' life consists of an enactment of one of the various social roles which change over the course of the life cycle. By contrast, the 'private' part of her self, her 'other self', represents the 'personal unconscious' and remains constant and unchanging over a large portion of the text.

The important point to note here is that the interpretive voice draws a distinction between the conscious 'public' part of the self, on the one hand, and the 'private' unconscious part of the self, on the other. Thus, '*I* acquired another self with memories and experiences separate from *mine*, whose existence was unknown to *me*' (p. 15). According to Fraser, from this point onwards, the 'other self' deals with the incidents of sexual abuse perpetrated upon her by her father: '*In future*, whenever my daddy approached me sexually *I* turned into *my other self* and afterwards *I* did not remember anything that had happened' (p. 15); '*She knew everything* about me. I knew nothing about her' (p. 15); '*Because of her* ... I was drawn to other children who knew more than they should about adult ways' (p. 15).

The issues of knowledge/lack of knowledge touched upon here are of crucial importance and are critical for the scenes that follow. Note how the interpretive voice begins to use the third-person pronoun to refer to the 'private' self of the personal unconscious – referring to 'she' and to 'her'. Note how such references are set alongside references to the 'I' and 'me' of the 'public' self. Here, we see a distinction drawn between the third person, the 'other self' who has access to 'bad' knowledge, on the one hand, and the unsullied public face of the seven-year-old child, on the other. 'She' was causing 'me' to do things. 'Hers was the guilty face I sometimes glimpsed in my mirror' (p. 15). Clearly, here we have a third party who has access to knowledge that the first person does not possess; we have an innocent 'I' in contrast with a guilty 'other'.[2]

It is, therefore, clear that the interpretive voice draws a distinction between the 'public' reality of the 'public' self and the 'private' reality of the 'private' unconscious self. Having already described some of the ways in which the 'public' self is portrayed to the reader, and having shown how such a portrayal relies on a socialist feminist discourse, I now want to look at the way in which the 'private' reality of the unconscious self is portrayed. In turn, I will show how this portrayal relies on a psychoanalytic interpretation of events – an interpretation evident within the 'healing' discourse.

Much of the 'reality' experienced by the 'other self' is presented to the reader in the form of italicized text, i.e. in the form of the unconscious voice. This is because the details of such experiences are not present to consciousness and, thus, are not supposed to be available to the narrative voice at the time of reportage. However, many of the symbols and themes that later become significant in terms of the 'reality' experienced by the 'other self' are also made available to the reader in the form of the narrative voice's portrayal of events in the early childhood years. These symbols and themes are associated with the child's 'private' biographical reality – they take on a 'private' significance in terms of the child's early formative years of personality development. Thus, within the domain of the 'other self', events are located in a 'private biography', as opposed to a 'public' social and historical context.

This is further evident in terms of the types of descriptions used to identify the times, places and people involved in events taking place within the 'private' biography. It may be recalled that events occurring in the 'public' realm, in the main, were identified by the use of official descriptions, e.g. dates and temporal periods were specified, and proper nouns were used to identify people and places. By contrast, events occurring within the domain of the 'private' 'other self', are described in what could be called 'relational' terms. By relational here, I mean that the time, place, person and event are described in terms of their relationship to a 'private', 'subjective' point of focus, rather than a 'public', 'objective' one.[3]

For example, a whole series of symbols are developed which take on a certain 'private' significance for Sylvia in terms of her personal and family history. When a lady in the supermarket plays with the five-year-old Sylvia's hair she remarks: 'What lovely golden curls, just like a fairytale princess' (p. 5). But these curls serve to connect the child to her Daddy who also plays with her blonde hair and tells her that he had curls like hers when he was a baby. And Sylvia's paternal grandmother, known as 'Other Grandmother', removes a 'pearly comb' from her own hair and puts it into Sylvia's, as if she were 'looking into a mirror'. '"You get your blonde hair from your father and from me . . . Just like a fairytale princess"' (p. 18). As the text progresses, it becomes clear that this symbol represents the theme of inheritance as it is suggested that the incest taking place between Sylvia and her father is a product of their family history. This theme of inheritance is also represented by the character of Aunt Estelle, the sister of Sylvia's father. Throughout the text there are vague allusions to the fact that Aunt Estelle and Sylvia's father engaged in an incestuous relationship when they were younger. More family connections are drawn when the child panics at the thought that she has to kiss her grandmother goodbye:

> Why this revulsion for an old woman's kiss? I do not know. I cannot say. *This truth belongs to my other self, and it is a harsh one: Other Grandmother's caved-in cheek is the same squishy texture as daddy's scrotum.* (p. 19)

Events are further located within the context of family history in terms of the spatial location of the life of the unconscious 'other self'. Just as people (such as Aunt Estelle, Other Grandmother) are characterized in terms of their relationship to family history, places are similarly described in 'relational' terms. Rather than locating events in terms of some 'publicly' identifiable place such as 'Toronto', or 'Hamilton High school', events taking place within the domain of the 'other self' are located within the 'private' space of 'my father's house', or more specifically, within 'a single room' of that house. Additionally, 'Other Grandmother's House' also comes to represent one of the 'spaces' associated with the 'other self' in terms of a comparison that is drawn between the two houses: '*Just as everyone is deaf at Other Grandmother's house, everyone is blind in my father's house*' (p. 21). The themes of blindness and deafness point to another important symbol; that of the ornamental 'see-no-evil, hear-no-evil, speak-no-evil monkeys on the radio console' (p. 9). These represent the family's turning away from recognition of the abuse, a well-known 'symptom' of incestuous, 'dysfunctional' families. Tied into the theme of inheritance are the interrelated themes of mental illness, death and suicide. One symbol which is important in carrying these themes throughout the text is that of 'cats'. This symbol is introduced as the father threatens the child in order to silence her about the abuse: '"*If you say once more that you're going to tell, I'm sending that cat of yours to the pound for gassing!*"' (p. 12).

Alongside the themes of decay, decadence and inheritance is the 'glamorous', exciting and 'romantic' aspect of the 'other self's' life. It is in relation to such themes that the influence of Freud's theory of the Oedipus Complex becomes most apparent within the text. Such 'glamour' is represented by the Lawson family, the family of Sylvia's schoolfriend, Lulu. Lulu's grandmother was an actress and both of her parents 'look like movie stars' (p. 29). Paul Lawson, Lulu's father, is a lieutenant in the navy. Holding up a silver-framed photo of her father in his white uniform, Lulu asks Sylvia if she thinks 'Paul' is 'the deadspit of Clark Gable?' (p. 31). She then kisses her father's photograph and refuses to go to sleep until she finds an old tattered handkerchief which has her father's smell on it. Sylvia is characterized as feeling jealous; she waits until Lulu has gone to sleep and then takes the handkerchief, pretending it is hers.

Links between the Lawson and the Fraser family are drawn on a number of occasions. Lulu's 'big white house on Delaware Avenue' reminds Sylvia of 'Other Grandmother's, where Aunt Estelle lives boarded up, the only difference being that everything is dusted at the Lawson's' (p. 30). Comparisons are also drawn between Mrs Lawson and Sylvia's mother. For example, Mrs Lawson does volunteer work, like Sylvia's mother, but Mrs Lawson, unlike Sylvia's mother, gets her picture in the paper wearing a hat with a veil. The significance of such connections becomes clear at a later stage within the text when the theme of the Oedipus Complex is more fully articulated.

For the time being, however, it is important to note that the comparison between Millicent Lawson and Sylvia's mother brings forth issues of mother–daughter rivalry, competition and jealousy. This theme of the mother's jealousy of her daughter is evident throughout the text and is symbolized by the mother's disapproving and 'scolding lips'. For example, when Sylvia's mother finds her touching herself between her legs, she strikes her across the cheek, shouting '"Don't ever let me catch you doing such a dirty thing again!"' (p. 7). In defiance, the child lies in the dark with her hands between her legs singing, '"Don't ever let me catch you!"' and twisting her lips like her mother (p. 7). Similarly, when the child lies on her father's bed being sexually abused she thinks that the scroll on her father's headboard looks like her mother's scolding lips.

It is extremely difficult to provide an overview of all the themes and symbols pertaining to the 'private' life of the 'other self', both because there are so many of them, and also because they are all inseparably connected together. The important point to grasp here, however, is the *way in which* these themes and symbols serve to locate the child's experience of childhood sexual abuse, that is, as a product of family history and 'private biography'. As I have outlined in this chapter, the location of experiences in this way is somewhat different from the location of events within the 'public' socio-historical context. Towards the end of the first section of the text, however, it becomes clear that the 'private' location of events associated with the world of the 'other self' is beginning to take over and predominate. For example, the final chapter, documenting Sylvia's wedding day, actually opens with the unconscious voice reciting the words of the wedding ceremony:

> *Who gives this woman?*
> *I do.* (p. 138)

The fact that the interpretive voice is usurped by the unconscious voice indicates that Sylvia's 'public' consciousness is being overtaken by her 'private' unconscious 'other self'. The person 'giving' Sylvia away is identified as the 'I' of the other self, the 'I' whom the narrative voice has no consciousness of; the 'I' who 'belongs' to daddy.[4] In order to buttress the image of unconscious determination in this chapter there is a cumulative repetition of symbols associated with the 'world' of the 'other self'. As the young bride walks down the aisle, 'As the organ swells, I see my shadow intensify' (p. 140). This intensification of the 'shadow', of the other self, is textually indicated by the page's swelling with italicized text (the unconscious voice). This leads to the closure of this chapter with the assertion that:

> *I will have no memory of the wedding ceremony . . . I will have*
> *no memory of the wedding night. Sexual initiation is the territory*
> *of my other self. She who would-not-wear-white has been*
> *summoned to stand fierce guard over her own secrets.* (p. 141)

In this way, we see that the segregation between the 'public' self and the 'private' 'other self' is maintained.

For the purposes of this analysis, the crucially important point to note is the way in which the location of sexually abusive events within a 'private' biographical history serves to produce a rather different description and characterization of events from that available within the socialist feminist discourse. This is most apparent in terms of the contrast between the narrative portrayal of certain incidents as 'sexual abuse' and 'sexual harassment' over the course of the first section of the text, and the re-formulation of those very same events by the interpretive voice. For example, the interpretive voice typically characterizes previously defined 'abusive' events in terms such as '*my sexual relationship*with my father' (pp. 15, 39), '*my incestuous relationship* with my father' (p. 120) and '*our affair*' (p. 39). Use of the terms 'sexual relationship' or 'affair' presents an impression of mutual, active participation in sexual events. This image of shared participation is developed through the use of possessive pronouns such as 'our'. Obviously, this provides a totally different profile of events from that found within the first section of the narrative, where events were tied to the 'public' context of the coercive nuclear family and the patriarchal system as a whole.

Conclusion

From this overview of the first section of the text, it is evident that Fraser does, initially, locate her personal experience of childhood sexual abuse in a 'public', i.e. socio-historical context. Events occurring over the course of her life are linked into the dominant ideological context of patriarchy. As such, children and women are portrayed as victims of that system, ultimately powerless in the face of economic and structural inequality. In this sense, *My Father's House* could be said to offer an interpretation of childhood sexual abuse which accords with that of a socialist feminist perspective.

Having said this, however, coexisting alongside this 'public' portrayal of events is a rather different interpretation in which both the victim and the event are decontextualized from their socio-historical location and recontextualized in terms of an inner, 'private' biographical context. This perspective, culled from an increasingly popular 'healing discourse', provides a totally different picture of the victim and the event from that encountered within the earlier socialist feminist discourse. In the next chapter I show how, within the second step of the psychoanalytic procedure, Fraser's adoption of a perspective which relies on the 'healing discourse' serves to exclude the interpretation of events offered by the socialist feminist discourse. In turn, we will see how this has further implications for the way in which Fraser's 'personal experience' of childhood sexual abuse is constructed.

Notes

1.   In a recent novel, *The War Zone* (Stuart, 1990), incest is similarly portrayed as an example of male possession and ownership. The daughter, Jessie, screams at her father:

> 'You work and you fuck and you load it with trinkets, property, children
> ... you get extra-daring one day, really charged with your own ... essence,
> and you fuck me.... (p. 196)

    As Jessie's boyfriend prepares for a confrontation with her father, Jessie's brother, the narrator of the story, informs the reader that: 'Dad doesn't want any help from anyone – he wants this fight for his daughter's cunt ...' (p. 176). Further examples of incest as a product of male ownership and possession can be found in commercial pornography where images of fathers clasping padlocks to the labia of daughters to 'keep them all for you', can be found (Tate, 1990).

2.   As I suggested earlier, such contrasting descriptions are also used in order to produce a distinction between Sylvia's 'real' adolescent self, and the 'mere' persona that the 'Appearances' self presented to the public. It is, however, important at this point to bear in mind that a distinction is drawn between the 'she' of the 'other self', on the one hand, and the 'she' of the Appearances self, on the other. For example: 'Though I frequently lost control of her (Appearances) I never lost *conscious contact as I did with my other self*' (p. 66). The importance of this distinction will become clear in Chapter 6.

3.   Of course, in actual fact, whether definitions are 'relational' and 'private' or 'public' and 'official', they are all tied to their context. Objectivity and facticity, just like subjectivity and vagueness, are culturally produced. Here, however, I am attempting to locate the uses and the textual effects of different types of description.

4.   The father's role in the traditional Christian marriage ceremony, 'giving away' his daughter, exemplifies the pattern of possession and ownership within patriarchy – of females as the chattel property of men (Brownmiller, 1975; Dworkin, 1987). In Walker's *The Color Purple* (1983) this fact is clear as Celie's stepfather 'gives' her to a prospective husband: '"I can let you have Celie.... She ain't fresh tho' ... she spoiled. Twice"'. Celie's 'spoiling' is the result of her having been raped by her stepfather.

Chapter 5

Step Two: The 'Private' Location of the Problem

The wizardry by which moral suasion is converted to causal necessity is a requirement of the polemic of psychotherapy, in order to convince the patient of the truth of the diagnosis. The trauma of the two year old becomes the excuse for the adult . . . because the hydraulic . . . metaphors convince the patient that his behaviour is determined by these circumstances. For we all, in some way or another, share the prejudice that determinism relieves us of responsibility. (Louch, 1966, p. 92)

Introduction

In Chapter 4 I focused upon the first step of the psychoanalytic procedure within Fraser's text, highlighting the way in which events were located, in terms of *both* a 'public' context on the one hand, and a 'private' biographical context, on the other. It was argued that locating the experience of childhood sexual abuse in these various ways provided different interpretations of the nature of childhood sexual abuse, which, in turn, has implications for the way in which agency, responsibility and blame are allocated. In this chapter, I focus upon the second step of psychoanalytic procedure in Fraser's text, namely *Recollection and Repetition*. Here, it becomes clear that the interpretive voice 'works back' on the first section of the text in a selective manner which serves to prioritize the 'private' location of the problem, thereby prioritizing a particular profile of the victim's experience of childhood sexual abuse.

Regression

In the last chapter, I pointed out that Fraser closes the first section of *My Father's House* with the 'private' unconscious voice. In the opening of the second section, by contrast, Fraser emphasizes, once more, 'public' aspects of the scene. Here, the past decade or so is glossed over as Fraser characterizes the early years of her marriage, career and the historical context in which they were situated. She tells the reader that, in the late 1950s, Toronto was a 'stuffy WASP bastion' but, nevertheless, it was the big time to her (p. 145). As the conservatism of the 1950s gives way to the passions of the 1960s, Fraser, as a journalist, travels across the continent, interviewing all kinds of people. By the mid-1960s, Sylvia is living with her husband in the Colonnade in central Toronto. She summarizes this period of her life as one in which she loved her husband and enjoyed her job. Both her personal life and her career were going well. She had a marriage of 'affection, mutual respect, some material wealth, shared memories, good friends' (p. 145). What more could one ask for? Indeed, 'For a dozen years, life was everything I dreamt it could be'.

This positive, 'public' frame of reference paves the way for our entry into section two of the text. Here, there is no mention of the 'private' sense of reality experienced by the personal unconscious. The significance of this absence becomes clear when we examine the narrative portrayal of events within this section. For, as will become increasingly clear, in this section, the 'reality' experienced by the personal unconscious becomes paramount – to such an extent that it begins to determine the course of events. Hence, the reason why Fraser does not refer to these events in the interpretive voice is in order to preserve the impression that knowledge from the 'personal unconscious' emerges spontaneously and not as a product of reflections on the past.

Within the narrative, depression is characterized as seeping 'like poisonous fog' through the cracks in Sylvia's life. 'Depression' is personified as an active, independent, psychological force. This impression is buttressed by onomatopoeic use of the word 'seeping'. Similarly, 'I become obsessed with the image of a hangman's noose. It's the last thing I see before falling asleep at night. . . . It fills my dreams. . . . It hangs before me' (p. 146). Here, the subject 'I' is passively constructed, by contrast with the obsessive 'it' – the image of the hangman's noose which is constructed in the active voice, and, like the depression, takes on a life of its own. The unconscious voice is interspersed into the narrative as a means of further highlighting the fact that the depression is uncontrollable: '*Though I don't yet know it, my maternal grandfather hanged himself, age forty-four, and a maternal aunt soon would'*. Mental disturbance is a family trait of the Frasers. Hence, the narrative deliberates the possibility that Sylvia may have inherited depressive genes.

The depression experienced by Sylvia forces her to regress; to return to an earlier stage of psychological development. This is indicated by a return to symbols and themes found within the first three chapters of the text narrating the early childhood years. For example, Sylvia is characterized as being *'lured by memories'*; she 'finds herself' attracted to childhood haunts and she visits these haunts with *'a sense of mission'* (p. 148). When Sylvia goes back to her parental home and searches through her father's attic, she finds disturbing pictures of a pregnant, Satan-like teddy bear that she drew as a child. Connections between pregnancy, suicide, death and evil are developed, as when she reports that in editorial meetings 'I . . . frequently catch myself doodling . . . when I look down I discover Teddy Umcline [Sylvia's childhood teddy bear] with a pregnant belly. His jaunty tie eventually transmogrifies into a hangman's noose. Full circle' (p. 148). Note again the passive construction of the 'I', in contrast with the active force of the 'memories' and 'mission' supplied by unconscious forces.

The major focus of the narrative voice within this chapter, however, is upon Fraser's writing of an earlier novel, *Pandora*. It is important to note that the process of regression is portrayed as beginning *prior* to the process of writing the novel. Otherwise, since the novel is about childhood, it may seem as if the regressive experiences encountered by Fraser come about owing to the influence of narrative, literary techniques, as opposed to being the product of autonomous psychic forces. Indeed, in order to further forestall this interpretation, it is made clear to the reader that, at first, Fraser did not know what she was going to write about in her novel. For example, she initially decides to write a feminist novel covering 40 years in a woman's life (p. 149). However, when she actually begins to write, she finds that she is not making decisions about the substantive content of the novel. Rather:

> *My other self has learned to type. She presses my keys, throwing up masses of defiant memories – stream-of-consciousness stuff. . . .* (p. 149)

As the 'other self' (the unconscious) takes over the writing of *Pandora*, Sylvia loses track of chronological time. 'Days melt into weeks. Weeks slide into months. Fall hardens into winter then lightens into spring' (p. 149). Danny informs Sylvia that she does not seem to notice that time is passing. Sylvia explains to him that the manuscript is over two thousand pages long, written in the 'first person hysterical . . . like a gush of primordial pain' from a part of her that she never knew existed (p. 151). She has not known what has been happening to her, and, moreover, she still does not understand. Suddenly, however, Sylvia realizes that she is *not* writing about 40 years in a woman's life, but eight years in a child's life. In all of this, the implication is that the writing of *Pandora* is not the product of a conscious decision at all, but the product of unconscious processes. Indeed, it is a 'classic catharsis' (p. 149). Although the manuscript was originally over two thousand pages long, 'one day in 1971', the book is finished and 'at 255 pages, it exists as an entity separate from me, *with its circumstances of creation still more or less a mystery to me*' (p. 151). Here, as I have previously argued in Chapter 3, it is clear that Fraser is simultaneously dislocating and locating the knowledge that she has used in the production of *Pandora*. By relegating the novel to the work of the unconscious, Fraser removes the book from the social and historical context in which it was produced.

At the end of this chapter we are informed of the date and place in which *Pandora* was published – Canada in 1972. After this, over the next three chapters (which comprise a substantial proportion of the book), there are very few 'public' temporal identifications. This is because we now enter an alternative reality; the reality of the 'other self'. Of particular interest here is the way in which an increasing emphasis on this aspect of reality necessitates a re-reading of the narrative portrayal of events documented in the first section of the text. That is, events which have previously been located within the 'public' domain (see Chapter 4), are now re-interpreted in accordance with the perspective associated with the 'private' world of the 'other self'.

The Return of the Unconscious

The very title of the next chapter, *Triangles*, points the way towards themes of the Oedipus Complex, family relationships and 'private biography'. The determinative nature of unconscious processes is made explicit from the very start with the statement that: 'It seems to be a law of human nature, as compelling as Newton's, that whatever is hidden in the psyche will struggle to reveal itself' (p. 153). More specifically, 'Through Pandora my other self had acquired a voice'. Thus, once more, Fraser emphasizes the fact that the content of her novel *Pandora* is the product of unconscious forces. However, *Pandora* is concerned only with the first eight years of a child's life. What of the 'other self's' knowledge of the years following this period? Here, the reader is informed that when Fraser tried to continue her story in a sequel covering her teenage years, she 'blocked'. The period was too 'volatile' to probe without grave risk of remembering. This notion of psychological blocking seems to be borne out in *My Father's House*, because, over the course of this section of the text (which represents the second and third steps of the psychoanalytic procedure), almost all of the major scenes are culled from the first three chapters of Fraser's text. Coverage of the teenage years is avoided. However, what is interesting here is the way in which psychological inability and 'blocking' is brought forth as a means of accounting for this lack of coverage. I suggest that an alternative interpretation, based on my findings set out in Chapter 4, is more plausible. Coverage of the teenage years is avoided, not because of the elusive workings of the mind, but because of the conflicting and contradictory insights that those years provide with regard to the interpretation of the nature of childhood sexual abuse. I will expand on this point later in this chapter.

For the time being, however, it is important to note that the 'agenda' of the 'other self' now begins to take over Sylvia's life in full force. What is that agenda? The reader is informed that it consists of the 'other self's' 'nostalgia' for '*her first love*'. The 'other self' now wants to 're-unite with daddy' (p. 153). Fraser elaborates thus:

> My other self required a daddy substitute, attractive to me as well as to her. The man she chose was, like most kings, married. This was not incidental. A triangle allowed her to hate his queen as a projection of the jealous fury she felt for the mother-rival who failed to protect her. (p. 153)

Here, the use of terms such as 'first love', 'daddy-substitute', 'triangle', 'projection', 'jealousy' and 'mother-rival' quite clearly correspond to the language of psychoanalysis. It is this psychoanalytic framework which sets the scene for the next important event in this section – Sylvia's committing of adultery.

Again, the language and imagery used here suggests a total loss of conscious control. For example 'When *the time* came to burst out of my marriage, it wasn't so much passion that tempted *me* but compulsion that drove *her*' (p. 154). Note how 'time' is nominalized here as an active, agentic force. This is achieved by making time the subject of the sentence through use of the determinate article 'the'. Again, we have the use of onomatopoeic words such as 'burst' and 'drove'. Just as the depressed Sylvia was at the mercy of 'obsessive' images of the hangman's noose, so too is the adulterous Sylvia at the mercy of 'compulsive' forces.

Throughout this chapter, in preparation for a scene where Sylvia commits adultery, there is a return to significant symbols and themes associated with Sylvia's early 'private' biography. Descriptions of persons, places and time are all reminiscent of the 'private' relational characterization of the world of the 'private' 'other self'. Indeed, it is not Sylvia Fraser who commits adultery, rather, it is her 'other self'. Moreover, the adulterous act takes place at the house of Sylvia's childhood friend, the Lawsons – a house that has previously been compared in the text with 'Other Grandmother's House'. As I argued in Chapter 4, Other Grandmother's House is associated with the themes of inheritance, decay and death. Perhaps most significantly, however, is the fact that the actual experiences of childhood sexual abuse are re-described here by use of terms such as 'first love' and 'incestuous affair'.

The narrative is concerned to build up links to past family history prior to the actual scene of adultery. For example, in a hospital scene (pp. 168–70), Sylvia, along with her mother and sister, visits her father, who is now old and infirm. This scene is clearly reminiscent of the child's weekly visits to see Other Grandmother reported in a very early stage of *My Father's House*. Indeed, this link is made within the narrative as Sylvia finds herself remembering Sunday visits to Other Grandmother's house. In the actual hospital scene, a connection is drawn between Sylvia and her Aunt Estelle, when Sylvia's father opens his eyes, looks directly into Sylvia's face and says: 'Thanks for coming, Estelle' (p. 170). Sylvia's 'other self' shrieks inside her, '*it's not Aunt Estelle. It's me!...*' (p. 170). Such connections are significant because, as I suggested in Chapter 4, there are continual allusions within the text to the fact that Aunt Estelle and Sylvia's father engaged in an incestuous relationship when they were children. The character of Aunt Estelle thus serves to advance the theme of repetition of past events within the present and, thus, to account for the incidence of abuse in terms of 'private' family history.

The process of psychological regression taking place in Sylvia's life is most evident in what could be called the major scene of repetition (pp. 170–2). Here, the fact that regression is taking place is marked by the dense interspersion of italicized text (the unconscious voice) into the main body of the narrative. This italicized text consists of selected pieces of text which are repeated from the very early stages of childhood. For example:

> Paul opens [the door] wearing a white terry bathrobe, his gray hair wet and tufted as if from the shower. *My daddy sits on his bed in his undershirt....* (p. 171 [6])[1]

And:

> Gazing into my eyes, Paul announces: 'Amazing! Wasn't that amazing? I haven't done anything quite so impulsive since I was seventeen.'
> *My daddy and I share secrets.* (p. 171 [6])

This consists of the technique of *redundancy*, to borrow an expression from linguistics, which involves the use of repetition in order that the author can ensure optimum reception of a message.

The adultery scene, as I have already suggested, is located spatially at the Lawsons' house which is connected with Other Grandmother's house: 'The Lawson house reminds me of Other Grandmother's house, where Aunt Estelle lives boarded up' (p. 30). This house is used in order to signify the return of the past into the present, and this fact is made even more explicit by the use of words such as 'antique', 'old-fashioned', 'tradition' and a 'shrine'. Within this scene, people who took on a significant role in the child's early biography are brought to the forefront. Thus, we encounter Paul Lawson, the father of one of Sylvia's childhood friends. He is the man with whom the adult Sylvia now has an affair. He serves as the substitute father-figure. His connection with the theme of the Oedipus Complex becomes quite obvious when the chapters in which he first appears are re-read. Seemingly innocuous references to persons, events and connections can be seen, in retrospect, as fore-shadowing, as building up fuel for the psychoanalytic fire. For example, in the first section of the text, Sylvia was characterized as feeling jealous of Paul Lawson's daughter, Lulu, when she kissed her father's picture and fell asleep with his handkerchief which had his smell on it. Additionally, in this chapter Paul tells Sylvia that he has not been able to get her off his mind. '"How do you feel about that?"', he asks, '"the father of your high-school chum . . . a dirty old man"' (p. 161).

Over the course of the adultery scene, and during the act of sexual intercourse itself, the 'other self' takes over and this is made clear by the use of italics (the unconscious voice). A point of extreme importance here is the way in which the actions of the 'other self' are characterized. For example, in this part of the text the unconscious voice uses language which is typically associated with a child. There are references to 'daddy', 'Teddy', 'granny', 'little girl', 'the trapped princess'. Behaviour is similarly described in typically child-like terms such as: 'babble', 'giddily', 'childish bravado', 'childlike'.

The characterization of the reality experienced by the 'other self' as child-like is also evident at other stages within the text. For example, in the opening stages of the text, Fraser points out that the 'other self' remained '*morally and emotionally a child*' who functioned on '*instinct rather than intelligence*' (p. 24). And in the process of writing *Pandora*, the return of unconscious memories entails a return to the world of childhood. Fraser tells us that:

> The deeper I delve through my time warp into the past, the more vivid it grows at the expense of the present-day world. It's as if I have fallen down the Alice-in-Wonderland hole into that detailed child's universe below an adult's kneecaps where getting poop on my shoes . . . [is a] serious worry. (p. 149)

And:

> As I write, the world inside my head becomes more real than the physical world; feelings more real than facts; thoughts more real than spoken words; my unconscious mind more real than my conscious mind. . . . Now, as I let go of the habits and rituals that anchor me to the here-and-now to explore the lost landscape of my childhood. . . . (p. 150)

As part of the portrayal of this child-like world, the 'other self' is characterized as having no real concept of time. She is '*feckless and impatient. To her, as to any child, the delay of a minute is like an hour, an hour a day, a day a year*' (p. 163). Her life is confined to a single room that might suggest the '*season and time of day but rarely the year or even her age*' (p. 218).

This characterization of the 'other self' as having an undifferentiated sense of time corresponds to Freud's characterization of the unconscious as having no concept of time. Within the unconscious everything is 'mere sequence' (Carr, 1986, p. 97) – 'flux' – a mass of undifferentiated images and sounds. Events occur relationally and rhythmically, as a series of repetitions or cycles – day and night, one season to another. Unconscious life is governed and motivated by the satisfaction of instinctual needs. There is no sense of 'clock-time' or 'calendar-time', of what I referred to in Chapter 4 as 'public' or 'Official' time. In this way, the realm of the 'other self' is characterized in *relational* terms, i.e. in relation to the 'subjective' focus of the child's 'private' biography rather than in terms of 'public time' (numerical identifications of age or year).

This portrayal of the time system of the 'other self' is similar to that described by the anthropologist, Wax, in his study of the different time perspectives and *world-views* of the Pawnee Indians, on the one hand,

and the Bible-era Hebrews, on the other (Wax, 1959, cited in Roth, 1963, pp. 96–7). In his analysis of the Pawnee mythology and way of life, Wax notes their lack of attention to accurate measures of time, describing their way of life as belonging to a 'closed time system'. According to Wax, this closed time system seems to be found in most 'primitive' cultures, and in many of the older civilizations that do not stem from the ancient Hebrew. Such a time system, as both historical and anthropological studies have shown, has a crucial impact on the way in which both individuals and societies understand relations between cause and effect. This, in turn, has an impact on the way in which agency and responsibility is attributed to people and events (see also Pollner, 1987; Elias, 1992). For example, Elias (1992) argues that the introduction of clocks and calendars into developed industrial states served to introduce changes in patterns of self-regulation which eventually led to a relatively high level of self-regulation and to the development of moral concepts such as individual responsibility and individual conscience (Elias, 1992, p. 24).

The development of the child's ability to regulate his/her feelings and conduct, and to develop a sense of moral agency and individual responsibility, is similarly linked to the 'learning of time' which takes place between the ages of seven and nine (Elias, 1992, p. 139). Prior to this stage of development, the child does not possess the appropriate moral resources by which to hold his/her behaviour in check. Hence, morally or culturally inappropriate behaviour performed by a young child is often excused on this basis. Given this fact, it is important to point out that one of the ways in which other members of society can excuse their own morally inappropriate behaviour, or the morally inappropriate behaviour of others (and thus diminish responsibility for action), is by appealing to a 'child-like' mentality. This often occurs in criminal cases in which the defence, seeking to prove the diminished responsibility of the defendant, argues that the criminal act was the product of an 'immature' mind. Fraser's portrayal of the act of adultery as an act performed by the child-like 'other self', could, therefore, be seen as an attempt to diminish responsibility for her morally inappropriate behaviour.

Decontextualization and Recontextualization

Infantile Sexuality

Responsibility for the act of adultery, is then, attributed to the 'other self'. As the 'other self' is characterized as child-like, however, this responsibility is, to a certain extent, diminished. However, it must be emphasized that this reduction of responsibility is not a *fait accompli*. This is mainly due to the fact that when a person is categorized in a certain way (e.g. as 'child-like'), this categorization is open to challenge. Moreover, the categories that we use to describe people carry certain 'in-built vulnerabilities' (Watson, 1978). For example, if I want to convey an image of 'innocence' I may find it useful to bring forth the category 'child'. However, this category carries certain 'vulnerabilities' because another person, who wants to challenge my portrayal of innocence, can do so by making reference to the very same category 'child', but by emphasizing other features associated with that category which undercut the image of innocence that I am attempting to convey. This 'in-built vulnerability' is especially relevant to the issue of incest and child sexual abuse, because questions regarding the 'nature' of childhood have been the focus of intense debate since Freud abandoned his 'seduction theory' in favour of his theory of 'infantile sexuality' at the end of the nineteenth century. Is the child a passive, innocent *tabula rasa* on which culture is written, or does the child have innate, active, sexually impulsive drives of his/her own? How far is the child 'innocent' with regards to incidents of sexual abuse? To what extent does the child participate, collaborate or even initiate the 'abuse'? I do not intend to immerse us in this debate. However, I do want to show how Fraser, by making use of psychoanalytic concepts such as 'regression' and the 'unconscious', is forced to take account of a whole rag-bag of contentious issues regarding the nature of childhood sexuality. It seems, therefore, that the attempt to excuse morally inappropriate behaviour by appealing to 'regression' and 'child-like' mentality gets Fraser 'out of the fire into the frying pan'.

For example, when Fraser portrays the act of adultery being performed by the unconscious 'other self', she is forced to address the question: 'Does this mean my other self had secretly enjoyed *her incestuous affair* with daddy?' (p. 154). This issue is elaborated on in what I call the 'Joker scene'. This scene consists of a TV interview between Sylvia and Gerald Nash (nicknamed Joker). Joker is one of Sylvia's old school friends who now works for CHCNTV, owned by Paul Lawson. Sylvia, after having published *Pandora*, is on a book promotion tour. The interview begins with a reading from a scene in *Pandora*, where as a young child Pandora is sexually assaulted by the breadman. In response to the passage, the following conversation takes place:

'Speaking for myself,' he smiles confidently into the camera, 'and, I suspect, a lot of viewers, I don't believe that incident for one minute. First you weave a false web of innocence around

childhood, and then you want us to believe—'
'But I didn't weave a false web of innocence. Pandora was
tempted by the cherry tarts, that was partly why she got into
trouble. That kind of detail is the strength of the book, as many
reviewers have pointed out.'
    Joker gives a pointy-toothed grin. 'Reviewers more gullible
than I, if you'll forgive me for remarking. For such a sexual
assault to take place, we must look at the conduct of *the child*.
Why would *she* get into the breadman's wagon in the first place?
Some little girls can be seductive at an early age. I think your
book is typical of the kind of hysterical imaginings we're seeing
too much of these days. According to you feminists, we men are
always the enemy.' (p. 158)

Here, we see how Joker accuses Fraser of bias with regard to her
portrayal of the 'nature' of childhood. Joker interprets *Pandora* as
portraying childhood as a state of innocence, as is clear in his statement:
'First you weave a false web of *innocence* around *childhood*' . . . (p. 158).
He then challenges this idea by questioning the traditionally assumed
connection between the feature of 'innocence' and the category 'child'.
Joker puts forward a different understanding of the nature of childhood
and, relatedly, a different interpretation of the sexually abusive scene
which took place in *Pandora*. For example, Pandora's presence in the
scene with the breadman is no longer seen as accidental or contingent.
Rather, for Joker, Pandora actually enters the breadwagon of her own
free will. She actively brings about the abuse. Hence: 'we must look at
the conduct of the child'; 'Why would she get into the breadman's wagon
in the first place?'; 'Some little girls can be seductive at an early age'.
    A crucially important feature of Joker's challenge to the child's
innocence is the way in which he uses certain categories to describe
Pandora. In the quoted passage above, Pandora is described in a number
of ways. These descriptions develop as follows:

1.   'childhood';
2.   'the child';
3.   'she' (Pandora);
4.   'some little girls'.

The first reference to the general nature of 'childhood' sets the scene for
the whole passage. This reference is made more specific in the second
description in which the determinate article 'the' is used. The third
reference uses the third-person pronoun 'she', making explicit the child's

gender. The final reference in this passage is crucial. Here, although the passage has so far referred to the specific case of Pandora, there is now a generalization towards other cases, indicated by use of the indefinite article 'some'. Note, however, that in this move towards generalization, we are not confronted with the suggestion that 'some *children* may be seductive at an early age'; rather, we have the statement 'some *little girls. . .*'. In other words, the noun to be determined *shifts* from 'child' to 'girl'. The significance of this move lies in the fact that the child's 'seductive' nature is established by reference to her gender. It seems to be the case, therefore, that the categorization of Pandora as a 'girl' is used as a means of placing some of the responsibility for the abusive events upon her. By contrast, as we saw earlier in this chapter, categorizing a person as a 'child' consists of a means by which one can attempt to claim diminished responsibility.

However, perhaps the most interesting feature of the Joker scene is Fraser's response to Joker's accusations concerning her biased portrayal of 'childhood'.[2] Rather than mounting a challenge to his conception of the nature of childhood (and relatedly, of the psychoanalytic perspective that his view represents), relying as it does upon discriminatory categorizations of the *female* victim, Fraser, in her attempt to display that she *is not guilty* of the bias indicated by Joker, accepts the terms on which his claims are based. For example, she denies that she has presented an 'innocent' version of childhood, and, as evidence of this fact re-invokes a scene from Pandora where the little girl is tempted by some cherry tarts. Bringing forth this scene serves a double function because it is also reminiscent of a scene in the opening chapter of *My Father's House* where Sylvia is tempted by her father's promise of pennies to buy candies from the sweet shop. For example: 'I count my pennies already imagining them to be blackballs and red licorice from the Candy Factory' (p. 6). Hence, by referring to the cherry tarts scene in *Pandora* as evidence of the child's sexuality (and lack of innocence), Fraser also makes implicit reference to the fact that she, herself, as a child, was not totally innocent. By doing so, Fraser attempts to forestall criticism by making clear that she has not presented the child as a passive innocent, and that she has not, therefore, presented a biased portrayal of childhood.

My real interest here, however, is not to decide whether or not Fraser actually does represent the child as 'innocent' or 'seductive', but to highlight the fact that her calling forth the 'cherry tarts' or the 'blackballs and licorice' scenes as evidence of her awareness of the issue of childhood sexuality serves to bring those incidents entirely under the aegis of the ongoing psychoanalytic schema. This has the implication that the contexts in which these incidents originally appeared within the text are lost from view. For example, the original incident, in which Sylvia counts her pennies imagining them to be sweets from The Candy Factory, is presented to the reader in terms of the exploitative context of the patriarchal nuclear family. For example:

Now when my daddy plays with me I keep my eyes tightly scrunched so I can't see. I don't want his pennies or his candies or his cookies ... I hold my breath to keep from crying because daddy won't love me love me love me. (p. 11)

Here, emphasis is not on the question of the little girl's sexual guilt or innocence. Rather, at this early stage within the text, the important issue was the fact of the child's social, economic and emotional dependence upon her father. The 'personal' or 'intimate' child–father relationship was tied into the 'public' historical and social context of patriarchy. The emphasis was on the father's exploitation of the rights that he has over 'his' child. In the second section of the text, however, these critical points of emphasis are omitted as the incident is extracted from its original context and used as trade upon the psychoanalytic market.

Similar points can be made in relation to the adultery scene described earlier in this chapter. In anticipation of criticisms such as Joker's, Fraser is concerned to display active participation on the part of the child-like 'other self'. After having sex, Paul apologizes to Sylvia for 'jumping' her as soon as she opened the door. Then he asks '"For the record, why did you come?"'. Sylvia begins her 'covering statement' but quickly breaks off. '"For this"', she answers. As we have already seen, the adultery scene takes place during the process of regression. This means that it is supposed to be a direct repetition of events that took place during childhood. Indeed, the text attempts to create this impression through its heavy use of italics. Given this notion of repetition, therefore, it is clear that the reason Sylvia gives for visiting Paul (i.e. for sex), also has implications for her 'visiting' her father's bedroom in earlier childhood scenes. The implication is that she also desired sex as a child. The important point to note here is that the focus upon childhood motivation or drive (a focus deriving from the psychoanalytic framework), fails to take into consideration the social context of the abusive situation. That is to say, by drawing a direct analogy between sexual events occurring within the adult world (between Sylvia and Paul), and those occurring within the child's world (between Sylvia and her father), there is no recognition of the different rights and duties and, thus, the different degrees of exploitation, evident within the two situations.

Love and Marriage

I suggested earlier in this chapter that this section of the text, which represents the second step of the psychoanalytic procedure, draws mainly on the early chapters of *My Father's House* which document the early childhood years. This serves to emphasize the determinative impact of childhood events on the course of adulthood. However, as part and parcel of this emphasis, I have also suggested that Fraser's avoidance of the adolescent years is necessary because the narrative portrayal of these years is very much influenced by a socialist feminist perspective which, in turn, may call into question the validity of the interpretations bestowed upon events by the psychoanalytic framework.

However, this does not mean that 'topics' and 'themes' covered within the adolescent years, such as love, marriage and mental illness, are not addressed in this second section of the text. Indeed, they are. However, they are addressed in rather different terms from the way in which they were addressed in the first section of the text (see Chapter 4). Just as in the case of 'infantile sexuality' the original context of events was omitted in order that the psychoanalytic schema could bring events under its own interpretive framework, so too is the case with regards to issues such as love and mental illness.

For example, in the second section of the text, compulsive, unconscious forces are portrayed as causal factors motivating Sylvia to commit adultery. Now, in order to present this portrayal of events as convincing, it is important that the reader should not be able to find any other reason to account for Fraser's committing of adultery. If an 'external' factor (such as problems within the marriage) cannot be found, then the act of adultery can more convincingly be seen as the product of 'internal', 'unknown' psychological forces. Indeed, this is precisely what Fraser tries to do. As I showed earlier in this chapter, Fraser constructs a picture of her marriage as one of contentment and happiness. Adultery is characterized as a 'large word' beginning with a 'scarlet letter'. The author tells us that over the course of 15 years of marriage she had never considered adultery. She had no need to because her marriage consisted of 'romance', 'fun' and 'glamour'. Moreover, her husband was her best friend (p. 153). This picture of the 'perfect marriage' is sustained both in terms of Sylvia's and other people's perceptions of the marriage. For example, prior to the adultery scene, Paul asks Sylvia: '"Am I being entirely absurd, or do you suppose we could have an affair?"' Sylvia replies 'rather starchily' that she has never been unfaithful to her husband, and, furthermore, that she has never even thought of being unfaithful. In a similar vein Sylvia's friend, Lulu, tells her that as far as she is concerned, Danny and Sylvia have got 'the perfect marriage' (p. 167). Immediately after the adultery scene, Sylvia returns home to Danny, who waits for her with a kiss, a bottle of wine, and a kitten – a present for their sixteenth wedding anniversary. Sylvia 'gags' out the words: '"Thank you, Danny, it's perfect." Like you' (p. 175).[3] When Sylvia separates from Danny she tries, unsuccessfully, to explain her reasons for leaving. In some ways, she ruminates, a good marriage is more vulnerable than a bad one, because the expectations are so high. Moreover, Danny 'deserves more' than Sylvia can give him. However, although Sylvia tries to find a 'good reason' that will account for why she left her husband, she is at a loss to do so. She ends up by saying, 'I left because I left'. All of this lends credence to the fact that the unconscious workings of the mind caused Sylvia to commit adultery. Hence: 'Like a sleepwalker *I* watched askance while *someone who looked like me* cast aside everything *I* valued . . .' (p. 154).

It is important to point out that the conception of love and marriage developed in this section of the text is rather different from that found within the first section. As I demonstrated in Chapter 4, there the experience of 'love' was tied into the economic and social context and, thus, themes of male possession and dominance prevailed. Indeed, given the fact that the break-up of Sylvia's marriage begins to take place in 1971, the historical period witnessing the emergence of the feminist movement and Women's Liberation, 'the beginning of a period when domestic conflict seemed just part of all the other terrible things that were happening out in the world . . .' (French, 1987, p. 573), one would expect the foregrounding of this type of feminist analysis. However, this is clearly not the case. As I have suggested previously, in this second section of the text there is a noticeable lack of 'public' temporal identifications as the alternative unconscious timetable takes over.

This is made explicit in a reunion scene in which Sylvia meets up with her old school friends. The women talk about 'the usual' – love and marriage. One of the women reaches the conclusion that marriage is 'a great institution for men but it sucks for women' (p. 178). Rather than elaborating upon such themes, however, Sylvia 'detaches' herself from the conversation and goes into the wharf for a swim. In this scene Sylvia is portrayed as increasingly losing her grip upon reality; she is losing control; something 'irrational' is taking over her life. This loss of control is made clear by her loss of temporal orientation. For example, as she emerges from the water, she asks:

'What time is it?'
'4.15.'

'It can't be.' I pick up my watch: 4:16. 'That's two hours, but I was gone only about twenty minutes.'
'The hell you were.' My skin is puckered and blue. 'It can't be!'.
(p. 179)

In another scene which takes place after Danny and Sylvia have split up the narrative touches upon earlier themes of male possession. As they discuss their separate lives Danny says that he is miserable living alone; all the plants are dying. Sylvia suggests that he may be over-watering them to which Danny responds with 'a wry smile': '"That sounds like me"', he comments. Here, it is implied that Danny is over-possessive and this implication is buttressed by his next question which is asked with 'clenched knuckles': '"Is there someone else?"'. Sylvia answers in the negative and uses this question as a means of deliberating further upon her 'reasons' for leaving the marriage. Again, the issue is diverted away from the context of male ownership and placed under the aegis of the alternative unconscious timetable. 'By now,' Sylvia tells us, she is sure she had to leave Danny but she still fails to understand why. 'Why? It makes no sense. Only that I am compelled. Why?' (p. 189). Here, it is apparent that Sylvia has a clear conviction – the conviction that she *had* to leave her husband, but she can find no grounds for that conviction. Her repetition of the question 'why' prepares the reader for a further search for those reasons. This quest for a reason, a motive, is necessary in order to show 'who' or 'what' is responsible for the adulterous act that destroys Sylvia's marriage. The question of responsibility is made explicit at the end of this chapter when the interpretive voice appears in the form of a third-turn (see Chapter 3). At 'one moment', Fraser tells us, her marriage was the centrepiece of her life. At the next, it was not: 'Someone – myself? – had turned out the lights' (p. 186). Here, Fraser rhetorically expresses uncertainty in her search for the person responsible for her marital breakdown. This is indicated by use of the word 'someone' – an unspecified person, and a dash, again indicating doubt and hesitation as the author queries whether she, herself, is responsible (i.e. – myself?). The question mark throws further doubt upon this suggestion, leaving the quest open for further deliberation. Of course, this display of uncertainty provides a means by which Fraser can, in fact, produce certainty within the text. By displaying Sylvia's failure to understand the motivation for her past acts, the interpretive voice is able to bring the reader into collaboration with its own authoritative interpretation of events. 'We', that is, reader and author, *know* who was responsible for the marital break-up, and it was not Sylvia Fraser herself.

Mental Illness

After the break-up of Sylvia's marriage, the text proceeds to display the onset of mental illness and personality dissolution. It is interesting to note that in this second section of the text the 'mental illness' experienced by the adult Sylvia is portrayed as directly comparable to the 'craziness' experienced during adolescence. For example, it is claimed that: '*As in High School*, I became a zombie while *her* needs, *her* goals, *her* secret agenda *once again* took over my life' (p. 153, emphasis added). As in the portrayal of issues such as 'infantile sexuality' and "love and marriage' (just discussed), however, drawing a direct comparison between early and later biographical experiences presents significant problems. As we have already seen, the main problem relates to the fact that the original context giving meaning to early experiences is lost. This, in turn, has a significant impact on the interpretation or the meaning bestowed upon certain events. For example, in order to come to terms with the significance of the statement quoted above, it is necessary to return to the adolescent years. During those years, it is indeed the case that a 'third person' or '*her* agenda' took over Sylvia's life. However, at *that* stage within the text, this third person does not refer to the 'other self' as is implied in the above statement, which draws a direct analogy between experiences occurring during adulthood and those occurring during adolescence. Rather, during the adolescent period, use of the third person referred to the 'Appearances self' – the social role relevant to that period of Sylvia's life. This is not merely semantic quibbling. It is a point of extreme importance because there is a clear distinction drawn within the text between Appearances and the 'other self'. This distinction is one of *consciousness*. For example, in the early stages of the text it is clearly stated that: 'I never lost conscious contact with her [Appearances], as I did with my other self' (p. 66). This distinction between consciousness of the Appearances self, on the one hand, and the unconsciousness of the 'other self', on the other, is important because each 'self' belongs to a distinct and separate realm of experience. For example, in the case of Appearances, this self belongs to the 'public' patriarchal world of the 1950s. By contrast, the 'other self' belongs to the 'private' world of Sylvia's unconscious life. As I have demonstrated over the course of the last two chapters, the way in which the experience of childhood sexual abuse is interpreted differs in accordance with the 'public' and 'private' domains. However, drawing a direct analogy between the two domains has the implication that the earlier socialist feminist interpretation, which is associated with the 'public' realm of experience, is lost as the psychoanalytic interpretation associated with the 'private' domain of experience gains ground.

The difference between the two domains can be made clearer by reference to some examples. As an adult experiencing the onset of mental illness, Sylvia suffers from increasing obsessions and delusions; she stares 'malevolently' at the telephone, willing it to ring, deluding herself with the belief that she possesses magical powers. The narrative explicitly suggests that Sylvia had the very same delusions as an adolescent, when she was 'just as crazy' (p. 180). Here, then, it is clear that the delusion is seen as 'belonging' solely to Sylvia and her psychopathological history; the delusion indicates some form of psychological maladaptation. This interpretation is imported back onto adolescent experiences as they are portrayed as directly comparable to the illness suffered by Sylvia in her adult life.

However, if one returns to examine the way in which such 'delusional' experiences were actually portrayed during the adolescent years, it becomes clear that these 'delusions' were not 'possessed' by one pathological individual. Rather, such 'delusions' were seen as a *collective* feature of the reality experienced by the majority of girls and women. For example, as an adolescent, Sylvia manages to convince herself that by staring at her prospective boyfriend 'whenever and wherever' possible, she will 'extract the desired invitation' to the school dance. The narrative makes clear that Sylvia is '*not alone*' in such practices or beliefs. Sylvia is characterized as having spent many a 'sweated hour' with her friends on the Ouija board, as they plead for it to tell them whether or not they will be invited to the school dance. Similarly, women at the 'Sparkling Soda Water Company' (where Sylvia works before leaving for university), 'dream' and 'delude' themselves into believing in the 'Right Man' and the 'Right House'; and female students at the University of Western Ontario queue to have their fortunes told. Moreover, such delusions and beliefs are connected to '*our* uncertain futures' (p. 123); they are the 'last refuge of the powerless' (p. 73). In other words, they do not consist of pathological symptoms deriving from the mental illness of one individual. Rather, obsessional beliefs, jealousy, craziness, self-harm, suicide – all symptoms supposedly pointing towards the existence of mental illness – are alternatively interpreted as the products of 'false-consciousness' deriving from existence in a patriarchal world (see Chapter 4).

Failure to take account of these earlier interpretations within the second section of the text, however, gives the impression that Sylvia has had an underlying predisposition towards mental illness and suicide over the course of her whole life. Other scenes are used to build up this picture. The reunion scene mentioned earlier is a case in point. One of the women mentions her obsessional jealousy of her husband's lover. This jealousy is located within the context of marriage – an institution that 'sucks for women' because it encourages relations of economic and emotional dependency. By contrast, however, Sylvia's 'obsessional jealousy' of her lover's wife is seemingly detached from such considerations. Her obsessions are the mysterious obsessions of the Oedipal 'other self', seemingly disconnected from the institutional context of marriage. The same can be said of her plans for suicide as she flips 'randomly' through her diary to the date of Halloween – 31 October 1973 – 'the festival of cats and witches' (p. 180). With a black pen she scratches out the date, vowing that it will be the last day that she will remain alive.

Here, the symbolic use of 'cats' transports the reader firmly into the 'private' reality of the 'other self'. Since the early stages of the text when Sylvia's father threatened to kill her cat if she told anyone about the abuse, cats have been associated with the themes of loss and death. Here, multiple connections between the cat symbol and the theme of suicide are built up. When the actual suicide scene arises, links to the past become paramount. Sylvia tells us that she has 'a plan' – a plan that she has been hatching 'for a long time, perhaps all her life' (p. 196). This gives the impression that her attempted suicide does not take place on the spur of the moment, but that it is an act that Sylvia has been *predisposed* towards. Note the way in which the narrative conveys an image of lengthy duration through the use of vague descriptions such as 'a long time' and 'all'. This continues when Sylvia informs us that 'for years' the image of a noose has hung 'tantalisingly overhead'. The narrative then lists the people in Sylvia's family who have previously committed suicide: her grandfather and her aunt. Hence, it is not simply the case that Sylvia is predisposed towards suicide. Rather, this predisposition derives from the rest of her family; from Sylvia's inheritance of 'depressive genes'.

This section of the text, representing the second step of the psychoanalytic procedure, closes with the continuing onslaught of images from the past – images that have previously remained repressed within the unconscious. For Sylvia, this results in many mysteries and quandaries that she is at a loss to understand. More specifically, this section of the text ends with the death of Sylvia's father. At the exact time of his death, Sylvia experiences a 'mystic connection' with her father which manifests itself in an 'unearthly shriek' which awakens Sylvia from her sleep (p. 202). When Sylvia returns home, her mother shows her a 'blond curl' of her father's, telling her that '"This was daddy's hair when he was seven"' (p. 205). Here, the 'mystic connection' experienced by

Sylvia is made clear as she grows 'dizzy' and has an 'overpowering' feeling of the uncanny. This connection is related to the symbol of 'blonde curls', which, as we saw in Chapter 4, brings forth the theme of inheritance. Hence, towards the end of this section, it seems as if Sylvia is on the brink of remembering the abusive incidents that she experienced during childhood. This, however, is preserved for the next section of the text.

From my analysis of the second section of Fraser's text, it has become apparent that the reader is introduced to the perimeter of the 'world' of the unconscious 'other self'. References to 'public' chronology are few and far between here. However, at the end of this section, with the narrative's reportage of the father's death, we are given some indication of the 'public' time period – i.e. 1973. The only other date appearing within this section of the text is right at the beginning with the publication of *Pandora* in 1972. Looking back over the events that have taken place within this section, such as the 'affair', the subsequent break-up of Sylvia's marriage, the break-up of the affair, mental illness, attempted suicide and the death of the father, it becomes apparent that these have all taken place over the course of one year. However, the text gives an impression that a much longer period of time has elapsed. This is largely due to the fact that, in this section of the text, we have entered a different 'private' time scale which bears little resemblance to the patterning of chronological time. As we have seen in this chapter, entry into this 'timetable' has the power to create a whole new interpretation of the nature of childhood sexual abuse. This is crucial because the interpretive work achieved in this chapter affects the whole course of the text that follows.

Conclusion

Over the course of this chapter, it has become clear that the 'private' timetable of the personal unconscious is beginning to dominate within the text. The evidence for this interpretation can be summarized in the following way. First, the portrayal of the process of *Repetition* involves a return to the early years of Sylvia's 'private' biography, that is, to the opening chapters of *My Father's House*. Second, the focus upon early childhood years leads to a neglect of the adolescent years in which a different interpretation of abusive events is provided. And finally, on the rare occasions on which events occurring during the adolescent period are addressed, the original context giving meaning to those events is lost, as their significance is interpreted in accordance with the psychoanalytic framework. In this way, not only are events selected which serve to advance the psychoanalytic schema of interpretation but, also, events that may prove challenging to that perspective are re-interpreted in a manner which transforms their original meaning and, by so doing, actually helps to make the psychoanalytic interpretation more credible. Having seen how this process actually takes place, in the next chapter I will focus upon how Fraser anticipates potential criticism of her position, and, in turn, how she actually deals with this problem.

Notes

1. Note that the second page number cited here, e.g. (171[6]), refers to the original point at which the italicized text occurred within the text.
2. I have placed scare quotes around 'childhood' because, as I have just demonstrated, it is not the 'nature' of childhood *per se* that is under issue but the 'nature' of the little girl.
3. Part of upholding this image of the 'perfect marriage' involves portraying Danny as the 'perfect' male. This was also made clear in Chapter 4 where I showed how Danny and his family represent 'reality', in contrast with Sylvia's artificiality and the hypocrisy of her family.

Chapter 6

Step Three: The 'Discovery' of the Truth

It was not the New World that was important – it might not have existed for all that it mattered. Columbus died without having really seen it, and, as a matter of fact without *knowing* he had *discovered* it. It is life, life that matters, life alone – the continuous and everlasting process of *discovering* it – *and not the discovery itself*! (Dostoevsky, 1955, p. 406)

Instead of a search for single origins, we have to conceive of processes so interconnected that they cannot be disentangled. Of course we identify problems to study, and these constitute beginnings or points of entry into complex processes. But it is the processes we must continually keep in mind. (Scott, 1986, p. 1067)

Introduction

Over the course of the last two chapters I have looked at the way in which the first two stages of the psychoanalytic procedure, *Recollection* and *Repetition*, are represented in Fraser's text. I have shown how, at various stages within the text, the incidence of childhood sexual abuse is interpreted differently owing to its location within different contexts – i.e. within the 'public' social and historical context on the one hand, and Fraser's 'private' biographical context, on the other. In this chapter, I focus upon the third step of the psychoanalytic procedure, *Repetition and Working Through*. So far, memories of the abusive experiences that Sylvia Fraser suffered as a child have remained locked within the domain of her unconscious 'other self'. The point of this final step of the psychoanalytic procedure, *Working Through*, is to bring these unconscious memories into consciousness. Indeed, the ability to call to consciousness events formerly 'belonging' to the unconscious domain is one of the factors determining the success of a course of psycho-analytical treatment. For the purpose of this analysis, however, the essential point of interest is the *way in which* Fraser accounts for the development of this knowledge. In order that an image of unconscious determination can be maintained, this knowledge must 'speak for itself'. As I will also show in this chapter, this means that it has to speak through the unconscious voice. To appear authentic, the final 'discovery' of the truth, like the build-up to this discovery (see Chapter 5), must be seen to emerge from 'internal', 'natural' forces which are not influenced by 'external' or 'cultural' factors. In this chapter I examine how this image of 'natural discovery' is achieved.

Passivization in the 'Discovery' of the Truth

The title of this section of the text, *Revelation*, implies that the 'truth' simply reveals itself to the author and, consequently, that her role in this process is minimal. Here, we are reminded of the author's earlier statement that: 'It seems to be a law of human nature as compelling as Newton's, that whatever is hidden in the psyche will struggle to reveal itself' (p. 153). Hence, it seems that the truth is not 'discovered' by human action, it is not 'sought and found slowly and with many blunders, but, being of divine origin, is whole, perfect, a gift, a miracle, merely communicated . . .' (Nietzsche, 1969, p. 57).

Throughout the text Fraser preserves an image of the 'unconscious' or the 'other self' as *owning* and *possessing* 'secrets' that the conscious self (represented by the narrative voice), does not have access to. For example, in the early stages of the text the authoritative interpretive voice often claims that the truth 'belongs' to her 'other self' (p. 15). 'Even now', the author tells us, she does not know the full truth 'of that other little girl' (p. 15). Before Sylvia can become well again, her other self must 'give up her secrets' (p. 211). How would she feel to 'discover' that the prize, 'after four decades of tracing clues and solving riddles', was the knowledge that her father had sexually abused her (p. 211)? Within this section of the text, when memories are beginning to emerge, we are told that these memories, 'belonging' to Sylvia's other self, are difficult to recapture because they have been 'deeply buried' 'inside' Sylvia for over 40 years. Here, the use of spatial metaphors such as 'inside' and 'buried', conveys an image of containment. This image is developed further through the onomatopoeic use of 'leaked' (pp. 15, 39, 66), 'seeped' (pp. 39, 146), 'haemorrhage' (p. 66), 'spewed up' (p. 94), 'throwing up'

(p. 144), 'gush' (p. 151), 'burst out' (p. 154), and 'stirring up' (p. 227). All of this builds up an impression that the 'truth' is located within a certain place and 'belongs' to a certain person.

As I demonstrated in Chapter 5, Sylvia is characterized as having no control over the actions of the 'other self'. This is because the 'other self' lives within the realm of the unconscious and occupies a different 'timetable' from that encountered within the realm of conscious life. Hence, if the truth 'belongs' to the 'other self', it follows that Sylvia will have no control over its emergence into consciousness. This image of non-control is buttressed by the use of 'vague' descriptions of time. For example, in this section of the text, Fraser tells us that she is approaching 'a time' when she would remember incidents that happened to her in the past. Use of the indefinite article 'a' gives an impression of imprecision and uncontrollability, implying that Sylvia's memories are lying in some somnambulant state between consciousness and unconsciousness. Hence, just as in the last chapter we saw how events were increasingly detached from their social and historical context, in this section too it becomes apparent that a similar process is taking place with regard to the author's 'revelation' of truth. 'My path of revelation', Fraser informs us, was 'the path of dreams' (p. 212). Once more, by characterizing the revelation as emerging from the 'private' world of dreams, the process of discovery is unhinged from the 'public' chronology of the social and historical context.

If, however, the act of revelation is related to the workings of the unconscious mind, why, after 40 years of repression, should memories suddenly emerge into consciousness? According to current psychoanalytic theory, one of the major factors involved in bringing to consciousness previously repressed material is the ability to overcome defence mechanisms (see Schegloff, 1963). A defence mechanism consists of an unconscious mental process which helps to avoid conscious conflict and anxiety. Typically, it may involve elements of projection – a process in which fear of a certain person or event is transferred onto an external object, or perhaps onto another person. For instance, in the case of Sylvia, a number of defence mechanisms were built up as a means of coping with the anxiety and conflict that the sexual abuse perpetrated upon her by her father caused her to experience. One of these defence mechanisms involved projecting her fear of the sexual abuse and her father onto an external object – her father's house. It is this projection mechanism which leads her to experience 'terror' every time she walks through his door. In order to bring her unconscious knowledge into consciousness, however, Sylvia must overcome such defence mechanisms. She is able to do this only after her father has died. It is only at this point that Sylvia can walk through the door of his house and feel 'not terror – a positive state' (p. 204). Only then does she realize that her father's house is just a house.

It is in terms of this ability to overcome defence mechanisms that Fraser portrays the death of her father as 'offering' her 'release'. For example, she states that: 'When my father died, he came alive for me. A door had opened, like a hole cut in air. It yawned before me, offering release – from what to where?' (p. 211). Here, it is implied that the death of the father played a decisive, immediate and catalytic role in the 'discovery' of the truth. This impression is reiterated in reviewers' reports of the text. For example, in 1987 one reviewer commented that: 'Three years ago, *following* her father's death, the truth slowly began to emerge from her unconscious' (Mackay, 1987, p. 3). This statement suggests that the truth began to emerge in 1983–4. Note how use of the word 'following' implies that the discovery of the truth occurs *as a result of* the father's death. However, if we actually look in detail at Fraser's text, we find that the father died in *1973*. The 'discovery' of the truth, however, does not take place until *1983* – a gap of ten years. The fact that this time gap has occurred is evaded within the text through frequent use of the type of vague descriptions of time that I have already highlighted. Drawing explicit attention to this time period casts some doubt on the catalytic role played by the father's death in the 'discovery' of the truth.

The vague descriptions of time used to portray events taking place within the 'private' world of the 'other self', however, suddenly change when the text moves on to pinpoint the actual moment of 'revelation' when the memory of childhood events returns to consciousness. The story of the 'other self', Fraser tells us, started in a 'blaze of discovery' on 'that April afternoon in 1983' (p. 218). Here, the use of 'public' chronological descriptions of time, coupled with use of the demonstrative pronoun 'that', indicate a relatively specific time period, especially in comparison with the vague descriptions of time used over the course of the second section of the text (see Chapter 5). The purpose of using such a specific description of time here is to mark out the revelatory moment as a truly remarkable, unprecedented and momentous occasion. This interpretation is supported by Fraser's use of a device called a 'contrast structure' (Smith, 1978, p. 39), which is evident in the following statement: 'The setting was banal, the circumstances unlikely for the revelation of dark secrets, but the time had come. I was ready' (p. 218). A contrast structure consists of a device in which an event, on the one hand, and the circumstances surrounding that event, on the other, are portrayed as anomalous. Hence:

(a) the setting was banal, the circumstances unlikely for the revelation of dark secrets;
(b) but the time had come. I was ready.

The first part of the contrast structure (a) provides the reader with instructions concerning the type of events that may seem 'fitting' to the circumstances. In this case, this is expressed in a negative form – i.e. the circumstances are unlikely for the revelation of secrets. The second part of the contrast structure (b), however, indicates that the revelation of secrets is about to occur, despite the fact that circumstances render this an unlikely occurrence. Here, use of the contrast structure serves as a means by which revelations from the unconscious seem all the more unmotivated and uncontrolled. Emphasis on the lack of facilitating circumstances implies that the 'unconscious' will work through anything.

Another way in which the author's role is minimized in the process of discovering the truth is by frequent use of the passive voice. This gives the impression that Fraser has no control over her own actions. Just as depression took over her life at an earlier stage within the text, now Sylvia is 'compelled' by an 'inner vision' that she cannot see (p. 212); she 'comes' to know the truth (p. 218); she 'approaches' a time when she will remember; and she 'feels drawn' to experiment with various psychological disciplines (p. 218). In all of this, once more, Fraser alludes to the force of the unconscious as a mysterious entity determining the course of her life.

It is only through careful, detailed analysis that some of the linguistic devices used by Fraser to portray an image of the unconscious as owner and causal agent in the production of truth can be brought to light. The same can be said for the broader, cultural framework on which the text is based, i.e. the psychoanalytic framework. As I have already suggested it involves three major steps: *Recollection, Repetition and Working Through*. In this section of the analysis I will concentrate in more detail on the third step, *Working Through*, which, in turn, incorporates a number of substages such as dream interpretation, abreaction and corroboration by a therapist. By working through this series of substages, *My Father's House* is constructed in a manner which shows that an acceptable procedure has been followed in the move towards truth. At the same time, however, it is important to note that because the truth supposedly derives from an inner, unconscious source, this organizational framework must not be made explicit. As I have already suggested, if the truth is seen to rely on external, cultural factors, then it appears much less 'natural'. This points to a certain degree of tension in Fraser's text. How can she present a picture of her knowledge as spontaneous whilst simultaneously showing how it conforms to certain principles of acceptable psychoanalytic procedure? This, of course, is not a problem unique to Fraser's text, but is a problem inherent in the psychoanalytic paradigm. In the analysis that follows, I will examine some of the ways in which Fraser deals with this problem.

Recovering the Discursive Framework

Dream Interpretation

In February 1983, immediately prior to Sylvia's 'discovery' of the truth about her past, she is admitted to hospital to have a hysterectomy. On awakening from the anaesthetic, Sylvia's body displays psychosomatic symptoms as it refuses to function and she is kept alive through the use of machines. Over the course of this period of transition, Sylvia experiences vivid dreams and hallucinations which return us, once more, to the symbols and themes associated with the child's early 'private' biography. Whereas throughout the text so far the meaning of these symbols has remained ambiguous, here, use of the Jungian method of analysing dream sequences leads to a gradual clarification of the meaning and significance of such symbols.

From within the Jungian framework, as soon as the personal unconscious is analysed, images arise which point beyond the personal to the collective unconscious. These take the form of 'archetypes' – images which have held meaning throughout the ages in dreams. For example, in Fraser's text, images of darkness, evil, blindness, Satan, priest, hero, magician, king, witches, caves, castles, demons, snakes, monsters and blindfolding predominate (pp. 212–17). Aunt Estelle appears, symbolizing connections between heritage and death. Symbolic images of doors, windows, darkness and blackness indicating the female genitals and reproductive functions also predominate (see Cox, 1964). An image of a 'black snake man' which figures largely in Sylvia's dreams, represents the 'shadow' – a Jungian archetype which is made up of things that are bad, and which typically appears in dreams as a dark man or woman.

'Blackness' and 'darkness', however, signal not only the 'bad' side of things, but also the beginning of a 'journey' (with all acts of creation there is 'darkness at the beginning'). Symbols of 'blindness' are important in the portrayal of this 'journey', because they highlight Sylvia's psychological inability to 'see', or to understand the significance of events which occurred in the past. In order to get well again, the 'blind person' must be made to 'see'. In this part of the text, the 'Joker' serves as a figure enabling Sylvia to 'see'. For instance, Fraser reports the following dream:

> *I am outside my father's house. A lawn sign reads: 'Home Truths'. A man perches on the porch rail, dressed in whiteface top hat and tails. There's something tricky about this man, like the joker in the deck of cards. . . . He laughs revealing pointy teeth. 'Someone who is hiding behind a blind is going to die, and someone who is blind will see. They are one and the same. YOU will see'.* (p. 215)

Here, the Joker symbolizes the Jungian archetype of power and thought, often portrayed as a magician. This archetype represents the power of knowledge and words, and the ability of such knowledge to achieve new life.

The crucial point to grasp here, however, is the way in which the significance of the dream symbols is made clear to the reader. In the text, dreams are conveyed to the reader in the form of the unconscious voice. As I have previously shown, because the unconscious voice uses the present tense, it gives the impression that the events taking place within its domain do so ongoingly over the chronological course of the text. Relatedly, this implies that the unconscious voice does not provide a retrospective perspective upon the past. In this particular section of the text, use of the unconscious voice gives the impression that the meaning of dreams derives solely from the author's personal unconscious. In reality, of course, the meaning of these dreams, expressed through the use of certain symbols, derives from Fraser's adoption of a particular framework. However, although this framework enables us to understand the significance of certain dreams, explicit mentioning of this fact is avoided, as the unconscious voice attributes the development of increased understanding to the vagaries of unconscious mechanisms.

The attempt to build up this impression is further evident in the unconscious voice's frequent claim that it already has access to the knowledge that is about to be revealed in the text. For example, at the beginning of the symbolic journey into the unconscious, the unconscious voice informs the reader that: '*In some way I already understand what is going to happen*' (p. 213) and similarly, the unconscious voice's use of mental imperatives such as: '*I must take this journey*' and '*I have to break the news . . . to both my parents*' (p. 215), are suggestive of mental and unconscious urgency. Of course, the unconscious voice's prior possession of knowledge and the sense of urgency implied within the above statements do not derive from mysterious, mental processes, but from the author's adoption of a psychoanalytic perspective with regard to past events. For example, the claims that 'In some way I already know . . .' and 'I *must* take this journey' both implicitly refer to the fact that the impending process of dream interpretation is necessary for the development of increased understanding within the text. Similarly, the claim that 'I *have* to break this news to my parents' refers to an important step that has to be taken within the psychoanalytic procedure in order that the patient can recover mental health. This is the step of 'rescinding projection' or overcoming defence mechanisms that I referred to earlier in this chapter.

Another feature contributing to the impression of unconscious spontaneity arises because of the juxtaposition of the unconscious voice's mental certainty on the one hand, and the uncertainty of the narrative voice, on the other. Amidst the unconscious voice's use of 'I must', 'I have to', 'I already know' and so on, by contrast, the narrative voice emits a proliferation of what Bruner (1987) calls 'subjunctivising' language. These include the use of first-person avowals such as 'I believe', 'I sense', 'I seem', 'I suspect' and 'I think'. For example, after one of her vivid dreams, Sylvia 'senses' that something 'real and important' has happened to her. She 'seems' to be on the verge of remembering something sexual having to do with her father[1]. As both Coulter (1989, p. 42) and Harre and Muhlhausler (1990, p. 100) point out, however, such language does not necessarily 'refer' to a person's pre-existent 'inner' mental state. Rather, such first-person avowals are used actively – they are used as a means of achieving certain practical actions in the course of social interaction. For example, the 'subjunctivising' language referred to above is used by the author as a means by which she can indicate her level of commitment to statements made at different stages within the text. For example, when the narrative voice expresses a 'belief' that certain things may have happened in the past, or a 'belief' that certain things are about to happen, then it is clear that the author is refraining from putting forward a claim to knowledge, i.e. that she 'knows' that certain things have happened in the past, or are about to happen in the present. This point is particularly significant given the different degrees of knowledge enjoyed by the narrative voice and the unconscious voice. One example of this is apparent in a dream scene in which, prior to the dream, the unconscious voice uses mental imperatives such as 'I must' and 'I already understand'. By contrast to this claim to pre-possessed, in-depth, inner knowledge, even after the dream has been experienced, the narrative voice claims to know very little. This is clear in the statement 'All I know for sure . . .'. Hence, by asserting a claim to mental certainty in the unconscious voice, and then contrasting this with an expression of uncertainty in the narrative voice, an impression of unconscious spontaneity is preserved.

The interpretive voice appears at the end of this chapter in the position of third-turn (see Chapter 3 and Appendix B). To recall, the interpretive voice normally opens each chapter and is used to preserve the meaning of events that have occurred within the previous chapter. When it is used to close the chapter as it is here, it also takes on this role of establishing the significance of previous events. The important point to note, however, is the fact that the author considers it necessary to provide more focused intervention than usual in order to maintain her interpretation of events. Here, for instance, the interpretive voice is concerned to make explicit the significance of the 'vagueness' encoun- tered within the narrative voice on the one hand, and the certainty of the unconscious voice, on the other. For example, Fraser claims that although she 'suspected' that something terribly wrong might have taken place in her childhood, nevertheless, she cannot simply leap from 'suspicion' to 'accusation', 'even in her own mind' (p. 216). Dreams, then, do not provide concrete evidence on which to base an accusation of childhood sexual abuse. Indeed, Fraser claims that she would never believe that her dreams expressed any 'literal truth', no matter how persuasive they might appear to be (p. 216). Here, it is apparent that the 'suspicion' deriving from dreams is characterized as unable to provide a basis on which literal truth can be established. Rather, Fraser's 'insight' and 'intuition' can only prepare her to remember (p. 216). Here, the foregoing narration of dreams is equated with 'insight' and 'intuition'. This reinforces the impression that the meaning and significance attributed to these dreams is a product of 'subjective' interpretation. In turn, this has the effect of evading the fact that the adoption of Jung's theory of dream interpretation has had a significant impact on the meaning of events portrayed within this chapter. After having relegated the 'findings' of the narrative voice to the realm of the 'subjective', we are then offered the possibility of attaining the 'objective' 'literal truth'. However, this 'literal truth' must be delivered from Sylvia's 'other self' (p. 217). Hence, the basis on which literal truth is to be established also derives from the unconscious. Here, the interpretive voice aims to preserve the impression that the 'literal truth' will derive from some private 'inner' realm, not from the following of organizational procedure.

Abreaction

After having established some intuitive 'beliefs' through the process of dream interpretation, we are now in search of the 'literal truth' which must be 'delivered' from the unconscious. Prior to the actual scene of 'revelation', Sylvia is portrayed as being totally disorientated in the aftermath of her hysterectomy operation. She is 'still more in the world of dreams than in the real world' (p. 218). As she lunches with some friends in a restaurant in Toronto her mind drifts in and out of the conversation. Suddenly, Sylvia's attention is caught by her friends' hushed, confidential tones. Listening to the conversation she discovers that Joker (the guy who interviewed Sylvia on the TV about her book *Pandora*) has attempted to sexually molest her friend's daughter. Sylvia reacts to this news by picking up her dinner knife, stabbing the table and shouting 'I want to kill that bastard!'. She then apologizes to her friends for her overreaction. Here, the narrative displays one of the signs used by psychiatrists to check that they have interpreted an event from the past correctly, i.e. 'strong emotional reaction'. Psychiatrists often stress the confirmatory value of strong negative reactions (Schegloff, 1963, p. 76).[2] Another related sign pointing to 'correct interpretation' is the 'flood of associations' in which new material from the patient's past floods into consciousness and corroborates the psychiatrist's inter-pretation. In Fraser's text, this process of 'flood of associations' is represented by repetition of parts of the interview scene with Joker in the form of italicized text. For example:

> My chest continues to explode as the conversation flows around me.
> *For such a sexual assault to take place, we must look at the conduct of the child. Some little girls can be seductive at an early age.*
> I get up from the table, almost upsetting my water glass.
> 'Excuse me'.
> *Did such an incident ever happen to you?* (p. 219)

In the presence of signs such as 'negative emotional reaction' and 'flood of associations', the narrative voice can justifiably make the claim that: '"I *think* my father raped me"' (p. 220). A further orientation to psychoana-lytic procedure is clear in Fraser's claim that she did not know what she was going to say until she heard herself say it. Only then does she 'think' it is true. Here, the narrative orientates to the importance of verbalization in bringing events to consciousness. This is why psychoanalysis has been coined the 'talking cure'.

Given that the stated aim within this part of the text is to move towards 'literal truth', how does the narrative voice move from its position of first person, 'subjective' and guarded avowal (expressed in the term 'I think'), towards a position of certainty; of 'objective' knowledge (expressed in the term 'I know')? This movement towards certainty is achieved over the course of the following three paragraphs as the unconscious, child-like self takes over Sylvia's body. However, this experience is distinct from other regressive experiences previously encountered within the text by virtue of the fact that it is portrayed in the form of the *narrative voice*, not the *unconscious voice* (as has previously been the case). This is highly significant because it demonstrates the fact that unconscious knowledge is being delivered to consciousness. Here, the narrative voice documents, in vivid detail, the child's experience of rape. This is achieved through use of the present and the present continuous tense as the following examples show: '*I am* sobbing . . .' (p. 220); '*I am* trying to shriek NO!' (p. 220); 'My daddy *is pressing* his belly against me' (p. 220); and 'My daddy *is forcing* his wet-ums into my mouth' (p. 220).

Over the course of two paragraphs, there is an almost exclusive focus upon embodied details. For example, reference to bodily parts such as pelvis, legs, shoulders, ears, mouth, arms, head, neck, jaws, etc., predominate. The text portrays the child's lack of control over the situation, as powerful spasms 'pass through' her; her body 'contracts', 'scrunches', 'snaps'; she is 'flung' and 'pressed' into various contortive positions. The child sobs without daring to open her mouth as the father 'presses', 'smothers' and 'forces' her into conformity. Here, the difference in power between the child and her father is made clear by the emphasis on brutal, physical coercion. The asymmetry in power between the two protagonists is emphasized further by the use of possessive reference to bodily parts. The bodily parts listed above are all preceded by use of the possessive pronoun 'my', hence '*my* pelvis', '*my* neck', etc. This is in contrast to the use of the third-person pronoun, as in '*his* bed', '*his* belly' and '*his* wet-ums'. The child's body is literally invaded as 'he forces me back against his bed'.

This vivid description of the 'original' scene makes clear the powerlessness experienced by the child in the actual act of rape. By portraying an authentic bodily experience, the text aims to give a tangible, concrete form to the 'dreams' and 'fantasies' that have comprised the focus of previous sections within the text. This scene aims to shock the reader by displaying the concrete reality of the abstract concept of 'rape'. This is clear in Fraser's statement towards the end of this chapter when she tells us that: 'These spasms do not feel random.

They are the convulsions of a child being raped through the mouth' (p. 220).[3]

This scene displays the step known within psychoanalytic procedure as *abreaction*. It consists of a process of reliving the past in the safety of the present. Memories are brought into consciousness, producing great emotional trauma while the traumatic incident is relived. The process is therapeutic to the degree that the patient is able to accept previously rejected material and integrate it into her ego as part of past history (Brown, 1963, p. 199).[4] This attempt to integrate is evident as the narrative returns from 'time travel' into the past, back to the present; back to Fraser's 'adult self', to her 'own Toronto bedroom' and to 'an April day in 1983' (p. 221). The narrative then proceeds to report that Sylvia is 'no longer the same' by virtue of the fact that a 'startling' piece of information has been fed into her head 'like a microchip in a computer': 'I KNOW my father raped me' (p. 221, capitals in original). Here, then, it is clear that the relived, embodied experiences lead the author towards 'objective' certainty. Moreover, it is this bodily experience that leads Fraser to a renewed understanding of events that occurred in her past. The re-enacted rape scene, on an 'April day in 1983', consists of a 'conversion experience' (Weintraub, 1975, p. 824). Similar moments of crisis can be found in Augustine's *Confessions* (the garden scene of August 386) and Rousseau's *Confessions* (the moment on an October afternoon in 1749 on the road to Vincennes). The essential point to note is that, at such crisis points:

> ... lives undergo a wrenching; personal matter in diffused suspension is catalyzed to take on clarified form; the personality gels like the crystal on its lattices. It is as if scales fall off the eyes which now begin to see purposes only seen confusedly before. The course of life is seen to have *connecting lines previously hidden converging now to a direction where uncoordinated drift and wandering prevailed before*. (Weintraub, 1975, p. 824)

Recognizing the impact of the crisis upon his/her life-course, the protagonist begins to perceive an order and meaning to his/her life, illuminated by the insights gained at the enlightening moment.

In Fraser's case, however, not only does she, herself, begin to perceive such an order to her life, but she brings in significant others who also now find it possible to gain a renewed understanding of events that occurred within the past. For instance, when Sylvia tells her sister that her father raped her as a child, her sister's response is immediate and spontaneous. She informs Sylvia that she 'always felt that something strange was going on' (p. 222). Thus, the scene of revelation enables Sylvia to 'understand' the 'mysteries of a lifetime'; 'shadowy deeds' that have always been 'dimly suspected'. These 'mysteries' and 'shadows' can now be clarified. Within 'a few seconds', in a click of comprehension, Sylvia's *understanding* of the past undergoes a radical shift. The narrative runs through many fragments of memory which have previously remained a mystery to Sylvia, but which are now prefaced with the statement '*Now I understand*...'. Thus:[5] 'Now I understand my hatred of my father...' (pp. 13, 103); 'Now I understand my childhood revulsion at sitting on his lap, coupled with a dim recollection that I once enjoyed it ...' (pp. 5, 11); 'the agitated child's drawings' (pp. 13, 28, 148); 'my fear of pregnancy' (p. 132); 'the obsessional affair in which I re-lived my relationship with daddy' (see my Chapter 5); 'the fear of confession which kept me from my father's deathbed' (pp. 201–2); 'the powerful psychic connection I felt at his death' (p. 202); 'the exorcised house where I felt not-terror' (p. 204); 'my sexually violent novels' (p. 211); and finally, 'my strange yet purposeful dreams' (pp. 198, 205, 212–17) (p. 223). Here, it is important to note that Fraser's text conveys the impression that the 'understanding' of the significance of these memories derives, spontaneously, from the 'knowledge' gained in the scene of revelation, i.e. from the 'discovery' that she was sexually abused as a child. It is as if 'understanding', like 'knowledge' appears in a split second, as a 'click of comprehension', in some 'internal' mental sanctuary. However, as Wittgenstein pointed out, when one uses the statement 'I understand', one does not refer to an inner mental process, rather, one uses a 'signal'. Wittgenstein expressed himself in the following manner:

> Try not to think of understanding as a 'mental process' at all. For *that* is the expression which confuses you. But ask your self: in what sort of case, in what kind of circumstances do we say, 'Now I know how to go on,' when, that is, the formula *has* occurred to me? In the sense in which there are processes (including mental processes) which are characteristic of understanding, understanding is not a mental process. (Wittgenstein, 1953)

We can tell whether or not someone actually 'understands' by looking at what they 'go on' or proceed 'to do' with their proposed 'understanding'. 'Understanding' can only be claimed when it can be shown that applied reasoning can occur. Even if 'understanding' is experienced as a click of comprehension one would still not claim understanding if one could not paraphrase, illustrate, expand or recast the phenomenon that one is claiming understanding of.

Given this understanding of the concept of 'understanding', what is Fraser actually 'doing' or 'signalling' when she lists her memories that she now claims 'understanding' of? Contrary to the text's portrayal of 'understanding' as spontaneously emerging from the unconscious, an analysis of this list shows that these fragments of memories serve to signify, or to build up a picture of childhood sexual abuse. That is to say, they cast an 'understanding' of Sylvia's case in terms of a 'typical' case of child sexual abuse. For example, experiencing an ambiguous relationship between love and hate, drawing disturbing drawings, fearing pregnancy, 'acting out', experiencing oppressive guilt etc. – all of these display typical 'symptoms' associated with having being sexually abused as a child. The most important point to note here is that Fraser, as both author and survivor of childhood sexual abuse, has worked with knowledge of these symptoms over the course of the text. This knowledge has served as a framework from which the author has constructed a convincing, authentic portrayal of her experience of childhood sexual abuse. However, in order to create a sense of mystery and suspense within the text, there has been a delay in 'tying together' these 'signs' and 'symptoms' within the narrative. Hence, when the various events are finally tied together, it appears as if they spontaneously and somewhat miraculously 'fit'. Our examination of the way in which knowledge and understanding are produced, however, enables us to see that the possibility of this eventual 'fit' has been prospectively orientated to over the course of the whole account.

Authorization and Corroboration

As we enter Fraser's final chapter in this section, the interpretive voice continues to preserve the conception of the unconscious as owner of the truth. For example, Sylvia 'finds' herself staring into her own cherubic face in a photograph of herself at the age of four: 'Tell me, little girl, what do *you still know* that *I don't know?*' (p. 225). In order to reach such 'residual' knowledge the author decides to visit a hypnotherapist. In doing so Sylvia tells the therapist that she 'believes' that her father sexually abused her as a child. Initially, this regression to 'belief', to the use of a guarded avowal, may seem surprising. Surely, we have already covered this ground? The reader has participated in the scene of re-enactment which resulted in the narrative voice's proclamation that 'I KNOW my father raped me' (p. 221). Here, this reference to 'belief' serves to downgrade the status of the narrative voice's previously exhibited knowledge. Why?

The purpose of this move becomes clearer if we examine one of the comments made by Sylvia to her therapist. She tells him that, so far, most of her 'regurgitated' memories have been 'physical and emotional' rather than 'verbal or visual' (p. 225). Previous memories are thus located within both a private bodily sphere ('physical') and a private mental sphere ('emotional'). Here, the continuing attempt to preserve the impression that Sylvia's memories have derived from the unconscious 'other self' who functions on 'instinct rather than intelligence' (p. 24), who closed 'her eyes so that visual memories were sometimes not recorded' (p. 218), is apparent. Such memories constitute the truth from the inner, the subjective, the unsophisticated, the naïve, the pre-verbal self. They are simply 'there'; they are not dependent, in any way, upon verbal, visual or cultural factors.

This chapter aims to move beyond the previously 'discovered' 'subjective' knowledge by developing 'verbal' and 'visual' knowledge as a means of corroborating such 'subjective' knowledge. For this reason, former 'knowledge' is reconstructed as 'mere' 'belief'. It is precisely through this juxtaposition of 'belief' and 'knowledge' that an unequal or asymmetrical relationship between the patient's knowledge and the therapist's knowledge is portrayed. Certain sorts of problems, such as child sexual abuse, require that a person seek help from a qualified counsellor or psychiatrist – that is, from a professional source. Such practitioners are qualified to deal with specific problems and thus have specialized knowledge with regard to a particular field. It is because Fraser orientates to this accepted social distribution of knowledge that she uses disclaimers such as 'I ask' and 'I believe'. In this way, she emphasizes her own 'subjective' and, thus, partial perspective as a layperson, in contrast to the supposedly 'objective' and authoritative knowledge of the therapist, whose function is to answer the following question: 'Did this *really* happen?' (p. 225).

The scene of the consultation with the therapist is of the utmost importance in terms of its positioning within the overall sequence of the text. This scene appears *only after* the 'subjective' revelation of memories within the previous chapter. It appears, therefore, as merely the *concluding part of a series* – a final touch that serves only as a means of *corroboration*, and not, in any way involved in the actual process of 'revealing' or 'constructing' those memories in the first place. This is significant because it suggests that the original perception of the problem derives from 'natural', unavoidable forces which the patient cannot escape from. As I demonstrated at the beginning of this chapter, the fact that knowledge of events is seen to be deriving from the author's *own mind*, without intervention from outside sources, serves only to increase the appearance of the veracity of her claims to knowledge. Indeed, this interpretation of Fraser's text is apparent in the following quote from one of the reviewers, which claims that:

> An amazing aspect of Ms. Fraser's story is her *spontaneous recovery*. She indicates having undergone some Jungian and Freudian analysis (learning, she says, how to interpret her dreams), but *in the end* ... she reports having her first recollection of childhood abuse *on her own*.... She *then* sought professional help from a hypnotherapist to recover specific memories. (Johnston, 1988)[6]

The impression that memories emerge spontaneously from the patient is maintained further in the pattern of interaction between the patient and therapist portrayed within this section of the text. The therapist is concerned to produce a definitive, 'objective' version of what happened in the past. His task is to answer the question that the patient poses, namely 'did this really happen?' In order to do so, he responds to the question by asking the patient to tell him what she 'sees': 'Now, tell me, what do you see?'. This consists of a 'perspective display invitation' (Maynard, 1991, p. 178) used by medical and psychiatric practitioners. Basically, the 'perspective display invitation' puts the patient into a 'voluntary' position in which it is made clear that it is the patient who is seeking help. This has the further implication that the role of the therapist (or the professional in question) is reduced to a minimum as s/he limits him/herself to a 'guiding role'. The fact that the therapist's role is minimized in this way in Fraser's text is apparent from the way in which his behaviour is characterized. For example, Dr Steven 'directs' Sylvia; he 'instructs' her; he 'suggests' to her; he is 'cautionary'. Moreover, he makes non-forceful comments such as: 'Are you sure you want to keep stirring up all these old memories?' (p. 227); 'Why not rest a bit?' (p. 227) and; 'Maybe you've had enough' (p. 227). In this way, these scenes exemplify a central theme within the traditional practice of psychotherapy – what Schegloff calls the 'Analytic Incognito' (Schegloff, 1963, p. 90). This 'Analytic Incognito' rests upon Freud's recommendations for the role of physicians. Freud claimed that: 'The physician should be impenetrable to the patient, and, like a mirror, reflect nothing but what is shown to him' (Freud cited in Schegloff, 1963, p. 90). The analogous suspension of the therapist's judgment and values within the psychotherapeutic encounter serves as an example of this 'mirroring' capacity. It aims to minimize the therapist's influence on the course of the therapeutic encounter in order that the products of that encounter can be seen as being elicited from the 'unconscious', *and only from the unconscious.*[7]

Hence, the therapist's role in this chapter is merely to guide the patient towards any residual knowledge that she has not yet had access to. Such knowledge turns out to be the fact that Sylvia was abused for a much longer period of time than she originally believed to be the case. Access to this knowledge is achieved by the therapist's initiation of age regression in his patient, which eventually leads to a state of co-consciousness, 'fusion' and 'integration'.[8] The use of hypnosis results in an ability to 'see' various parts of the self:

> ... my hands strike something solid – another mirror ... this time it's the mirror from my attic bedroom with two sides that tilt inward to create a multiple reflection ... I see a five-year-old child with matted hair and blue fangs staring back at me.... Before my eyes the child grows older. Now she is eight, nine, ten, eleven ... now ... now ... now ... now.... All three of us – my adult self, the blue-fanged child, the gaudy teenager – are reflected in the triple mirror. (p. 228)

Hence, it is the narrative voice's ability to 'see' various parts of the self that she had previously remained unconscious of, and hence 'blind' to, that enables her to move towards 'complete' knowledge and eventual unity.

Conclusion

In this and the preceding chapters, I have attempted to bring to the forefront the cultural framework used by Fraser as a means of developing her 'personal truth'. This does not mean that I am denying or degrading that 'truth' or 'experience' *per se*. Nor does it mean that I am attempting to deny subjugated persons 'a voice'. More accurately, and also more usefully, I am challenging a deeply embedded cultural assumption which leads people to believe that it is possible to have access to some essential, inherent 'personal experience' or, relatedly, to some singular, unmediated 'voice'. 'Subjectivity' does not exist in a vacuum. The interpretations that people give to certain experiences and events are heavily influenced by the cultural environments in which they live. Recognition of the impact of cultural factors on the production of experiential knowledge claims enables us to *locate* conclusions, explanations and the like within a *public* domain of knowledge. Possible 'problems' or disagreements can then be logically and conceptually subjected to scrutiny. This is not the case with knowledge claims that are presented as the product of an elusive psychological truth. It is perhaps pertinent to note that it is under the guise of the rhetoric of truth that some of the most terrible acts can (and have) been justified. This will become increasingly clear over the course of the next two chapters when we realize that the rhetoric of subjective truth actively encourages us to swallow a discursive pill that turns out to be no more than a palliative. This discursive pill is the 'medication' provided by the contemporary 'healing discourse'.

Notes

1. Here, we have recourse to one of the first of a number of signs that psychiatrists look for in ascertaining whether or not the interpretations they have offered of 'unconscious content' are correct – that of 'intellectual recognition' (Schegloff, 1963, p. 75). Here, use of the verb 'seem', like 'think' or 'believe' creates the impression of a semi-conscious state, a transition between consciousness and unconsciousness – a transition indicating, in Ryle's cogent terms, 'a noteworthy nebulousness' (Ryle, 1949, p. 150) – a vagueness leaving room for further clarification.

2. 'If a patient gets upset or angry about an interpretation, this is usually indicative of its being correct or at least in the immediate neighbourhood of correctness. Otherwise, the patient would not react so strongly to the interpretation' (Beck, cited in Schegloff, 1963).

3. As an aside, it is useful to look at the way in which the victim is described here. It is important to note that this part of the text aims to show the objective reality of rape in order that the narrative can proceed towards 'knowledge', as opposed to 'mere' belief. Given this, the victim is described in a 'pure' way, i.e. by only making use of the category 'child' as '*a child*'. This categorization enables us to see the *victim as a victim*. This is in contrast with earlier descriptions of the victim as an active participant in the 'sexual relationship'. As I showed in Chapter 5, this comes about by categorizing the victim as a 'little girl', i.e. by drawing on *both* of the category devices 'stage of life' (i.e. 'child') and 'gender' (i.e. 'girl'). Thus, by avoiding any reference to the child's gender, the possibility of re-categorizing the event from an asymmetrical encounter to a shared, participatory event is forestalled.

4. Typically, this occurs within the context of the therapeutic relationship and the corresponding processes of transference and counter-transference.

5. The page numbers in brackets after each fragment refer to the original point at which each fragment appeared within the text.

6. Here, it is clear that the failure to acknowledge the impact of the psychoanalytic framework on Fraser's 'discovery' of the truth leaves aside significant factors and circumstances which may alter the meaning of certain events. The fact that the author is well versed in psychological theories and therapies does not mean that her 'discovery' is not *true*. However, acknowledgment of the impact played by certain theories on the construction of the truth does provide a foothold by which one can assess, and if need be, criticize the (social and moral) implications arising from the appropriation of such theories.

7. Of course, this notion of the 'Analytic Incognito', as specifically related to the practice of psychoanalysis and psychotherapy, can also be expanded to include a

whole host of domains in which knowledge is produced. It is simply another way of speaking about the way in which we all routinely 'lose' the grounding upon which our claims to knowledge are based and, thus, of how we 'lose' the 'work' of reality production (see Chapter 1).

8. As Hacking observes: 'Integration, synthesis and fusion are the watchwords of modern therapy' (Hacking, 1991a, p. 857).

Chapter 7

Allocating Blame: The Collusive Mother and the Deviant Father

But, Gentlemen of the jury, profound as psychology is, it is still a double-edged weapon ... I have purposely resorted to the aid of psychology, gentlemen of the jury, to show clearly that you can prove anything by it. (Dostoevsky, *The Brothers Karamazov* 1958, pp. 857–9)

Introduction

The implications of Fraser's adoption of the psychoanalytic discourse as a means of making sense of her 'personal experience' become most apparent in the final section of *My Father's House*. This section is called *Resolution*. Here, Fraser examines the actions of her mother and father. In accounting for her parents' behaviour, Fraser adopts a psychoanalytic perspective which is characteristic of the later stages in her book – that is, of those stages representing the second and third steps of the psychoanalytic procedure (see Chapters 5 and 6). Interpreting the actions of her parents by reference to this perspective, correspondingly, involves reducing the focus upon the social and historical milieu in which the parents' actions were originally placed in the first section of the text (see Chapter 4). Of course, this involves making relevant a particular 'moral profile' of the parents' action – a profile corresponding to the type of psychoanalytical explanations found within later stages of the text. In this chapter I will look at some of the consequences of applying such modes of explanation to the parents' behaviour.

Establishing the Problem

In this chapter, we examine the way in which Fraser establishes the fact that her parents' behaviour constitutes a problem in the first place. Basically, the behaviour of Sylvia's parents is seen as 'deviant' because Sylvia, her mother and her father belong to the Membership Category Device (MCD) known as 'Family' (see Appendix A). This Device serves as a means by which the population can be divided up into members of team-like units or family units. Each 'unit' is expected to engage in certain types of activities which are conventionally associated with 'family' membership. These include activities such as 'sticking together', 'being loyal to one another' etc. In addition, the MCD 'Family' incorporates a number of 'Relational Pairs' (see Appendix A), such as 'mother–child', 'brother–sister', 'father–daughter', etc. The types of conventional activities associated with the MCD 'Family' 'spill over' into the relational pairs associated with that device. Hence, a brother and a sister are expected to be loyal to one another, and a father and daughter are expected to 'stick together'. However, there are also conventional prohibitions associated with family activities. One of the most prevalent of these in contemporary western society is the prohibition of sexual activity between parents and children.

In part, it is the fact that Fraser's parents 'breach' the special ties that exist between 'parent' and 'child', which makes their behaviour seem 'deviant' or 'out of the ordinary'. Somewhat ironically, however, when discussing the actions of the father, it is by reference to the relationship between 'father' and 'child' that the 'deviant' nature of his acts can be reduced and, accordingly, be portrayed as morally justified. I will return to this issue in more detail later in this chapter. For the time being, however, it is sufficient to note that Fraser considers the actions of her mother and father in two separate chapters entitled *My Mother* and *My Father* respectively. In accordance with the chronology of *My Father's House*, I will deal first with Fraser's analysis of her mother, and second with her analysis of her father.

The Mother

Category Bound Knowledge

The title of this chapter, *My Mother*, makes use of a possessive pronoun 'my' in combination with the category 'mother'. As I have just suggested, this category belongs to the MCD 'Family', which, in turn, brings forth certain conventional obligations and expectations. Research in conversation analysis has shown that, when a possessive pronoun is used in combination with a MCD such as 'Family', this consists of a very powerful technique for performing certain practical actions such as allocating blame and apportioning responsibility (Watson, 1987). In this case, the combination enables Fraser to 'count herself' as part of the relational pair 'mother–daughter' – and, thus, to bring forth some of the conventions, rights, duties, obligations and expectations associated with that relationship.

As Fraser casts herself into the role of 'daughter', however, she is confronted with the moral dilemma of whether or not to confront her mother with her recently acquired knowledge that she was sexually abused as a child. Her mother is now 83 years old. 'Logic and humanity', Fraser tells us, demanded that she would have no 'need' for such 'desperate information'. However, once more, Fraser characterizes her actions as uncontrollable as she informs the reader of 'a powerful *need*', an '*impulse*' and a '*desire* to confide'. Eventually, these 'subjective' forces 'articulate themselves' into an 'internal gush' of words. Here again, use of the passive voice serves to diminish the author's control over her own actions. This is buttressed by the statement that it is 'not I' who feels the 'powerful need' to tell mother, but 'the damaged child in me'. This, supposedly, is her last act: 'the need to tell mommy' (p. 231). Here, Fraser's bringing forth of her childhood status is reminiscent of the adultery scene (see Chapter 5), in that the author uses similar strategies in order to diminish her responsibility for her actions. It is not simply coincidental that Sylvia decides to inform her mother about the abuse in her childhood home – in her father's house. Indeed, Fraser characterizes this as a return to the scene 'of the crime'. Such details serve to reinforce the protagonist's childhood status and to emphasize the determinative impact of past events upon the present.

As Fraser casts herself into childhood status, not only does she diminish responsibility for her own actions, but, in the process of so doing, she also facilitates the task of making a complaint against her mother. This is because she is able, by calling forth the relational pair 'mother–child', to present herself as heir to certain entitlements based on our common-sense knowledge of this relationship. Thus, Fraser asks: '"Mother, why didn't you protect me?"'. This direct question establishes a standard of conduct expected of a mother. The activity of 'protection' can be seen as a 'category-tied activity'. Basically, this means that if a person belonging to a certain category (such as 'mother'), does not perform the type of activity 'tied' to that category (such as 'protection'), then the absence of such activity may be noticed, and may need to be accounted for in order to explain why the relevant activity was not performed. Indeed, this is exactly what happens here as the mother is portrayed as having failed to fulfil her maternal obligations and duties.

However, it is important to note that it is only possible for Fraser to accuse her mother of 'lack of protection' from her authoritative, retrospective standpoint. From this standpoint, Fraser assumes that her mother had access, at the time when the abusive acts were actually taking place, to the same knowledge that she, herself, now has. Any suggestion that the mother may not have had access to such knowledge is not entertained. Fraser speculates on the fact that 'the walls of her father's house were thin' and poses the rhetorical question: '*How could you not know?*' (p. 231). Here, in principle (I say in principle advisedly, as will become clear) is an example of *over-attribution*.

Jayussi (1984) elaborates on the related problems of under- and over-attribution by drawing on the way in which people make sense of actions and events in the course of their everyday practical and moral reasoning. For instance, she presents the following statement as an example of over-attribution: 'The woman poisoned the whole family'. In this case, the actual reality of the situation is that the woman in question pumped contaminated water into the house tank, which led other members of the family to drink contaminated water and, thus, to their being poisoned. However, if the woman did not *know* or have reason to suspect that the water was poisoned, it is clear that she cannot be said to have 'poisoned' the family without providing further clarification with regard to the circumstances surrounding the event. To say of this woman simply that 'She poisoned them', would be considered misleading because such a statement *suppresses crucially relevant detail from the description of the action*. Such details would have the capacity to transform the very *nature* of the woman's act. For example, a leaflet dropped through the door informing the household of the fact that the water was contaminated may have been eaten by the dog before anyone had a chance to read it. In this case, the woman was denied access to information regarding the water's contamination. To describe her action as having 'poisoned' the whole family, therefore, would be to over-attribute not only knowledge, but also intention and responsibility to the woman.

The same considerations can be applied to Fraser's description of her mother's action. By accusing her mother of failing to protect her as a child, Fraser implies that her mother actively (i.e. intentionally) failed to perform 'protective' activities. Clearly, however, if the mother did not *know* or have any reason to suspect that her child was being sexually abused, then Fraser is over-attributing knowledge and intention to her with regard to these matters. If it is the case that Sylvia's mother did not have any knowledge or reason to suspect that abuse was taking place, then, according to Jayussi's argument, she *cannot be said not to have protected* the child. At this point, however, it is important to note that this argument breaks down in relation to cases such as Fraser's. For, quite clearly, despite the fact that the mother may not have had access to such knowledge, she *can* still be held responsible for her failure to protect her child. This is because of the strong tie existing between certain categories and certain activities, such as that between 'mother' and 'protection'. Although knowledge of the abuse is required in order that the mother can 'protect' her child, the absence of such knowledge is not conventionally seen as an adequate 'excuse'. This, in turn, is because certain knowledge is 'requiredly possessed' by members of some categories (see Sharrock, 1974). Both Fraser and her readers draw on their common-sense knowledge that the mother, *by virtue of being a mother, ought* to have known about the fact that her child was being sexually abused. It is with reference to such socially organized knowledge that the question of whether or not the mother did actually have knowledge of the abuse is rendered irrelevant. She *should* have known and the inquiry proceeds on the basis of this assumption. Of course, such morally steeped assumptions comprise the very fibre of our practical and moral reasoning about the world and, relatedly, of how we allocate blame and responsibility. More specifically, such assumptions lie behind the 'mother-blaming' attitude so prevalent in childhood sexual abuse cases, a phenomenon highlighted in recent years by feminist researchers.

Locating the Problem: The Mother's 'Private' Biography

Working from the assumption that her mother knew about the abuse, it is necessary for Fraser to account for her mother's reasons for having failed to protect her. Hence, the text proceeds to search for the grounds on which her mother's failure to protect can be based. In the first instance, this involves recourse to symbols and themes associated with the psychoanalytic framework. For instance, the theme of the Oedipus Complex is brought forth at this stage within the text. Fraser character-izes herself as having been 'the other woman' who shared her father's bed, before she was five years old. 'Did some of *the wronged and jealous wife* in you respond to the gall of that?' (p. 231), she asks her mother rhetorically. Building upon this interpretation of events, Fraser asserts her 'suspicion' that far more than aesthetics was at stake in the 'battles' that took place over her flaxen curls – 'How you yanked at them, taking control of them', she comments. These reflections lead Fraser to suggest that such acts provide evidence for the fact that her mother was acting in the same way as a 'wronged and jealous wife' would respond to her husband's lover. Her mother's 'yanking at her curls' is performed by 'the witch in you, the Witch Who Knew' (p. 231). Here, it is interesting to note that out of 30 different descriptions of the mother in this chapter, only two are preceded by the determiner 'the'. For example, we have '*the* wronged and jealous wife' and '*the* Witch Who Knew'. These two references appear as absolute certainties within the text, thus corroborating the fact that the mother undoubtedly knew about the abuse. It is also important to point out that our understanding of the significance of these descriptions remains dependent upon the underlying pattern of the psychoanalytic framework.

As I have been arguing throughout this study, the way in which people are described and categorized is of extreme importance. People can be categorized in a variety of ways and whether or not a certain way of categorizing a person is appropriate or inappropriate remains dependent upon the particular situation. This means that people are routinely faced with the problem of deciding which category is appropriate in any given context. In Fraser's case, choosing the description 'wife' in order to categorize her mother on the one hand, and 'other woman' in order to categorize herself, on the other hand, is important. This is because, so far in this chapter, attention has been focused upon the relationship between 'mother' and 'child'. Here, however, attention is re-focused onto the relationship between 'wife' and 'other woman'. Clearly, this 'relational pair' does not belong to the MCD 'Family' as the 'mother–child' relationship does. Rather, the relevant MCD for the relational pair 'wife–other woman' would be something like 'parties to an affair'. As I have already suggested, a MCD has certain activities, rights, duties and obligations associated with it. In the case of 'Family' these would include 'loyalty', 'protection','mutual help', etc. Clearly, however, by bringing forth the MCD 'parties to an affair' different activities such as competition, rivalry, back-biting, etc. would be expected. The interpretive framework changes completely.

It is the interpretive framework associated with the MCD 'parties to an affair' which serves to provide 'reasons' for the mother's failure to protect her child. Such reasons include the wife's jealousy of the 'sexual relationship' that the 'other woman' 'shares' with her husband. Hence, the mother can be said to have 'special motives' which prevented her from taking steps to protect her child. It is also important to note, however, that categorizing the mother as a 'wronged and jealous wife' cannot easily be separated from her 'other' status as a 'mother'. This fact points to a potential conflict which may exist in a person belonging to both the categories 'wife' and 'mother'. For example, certain obligations (such as loyalty) are associated with the 'husband-wife' relationship. Similarly, certain obligations (such as protection), are associated with the 'mother–child' relationship. If the obligations of 'loyalty' and 'protection' conflict, how does the 'mother–wife' attend to both sets of obligations? This conflict (and others like it), are often resolved by establishing an 'order of precedence' as to which 'identity' is most relevant, or most important, on any particular occasion of interaction. Judgments regarding such 'relevance' or 'importance' are often challenged at a later date if problems arise (as is the case here). For instance, Fraser challenges her mother for giving precedence to her identity as a 'wife' – moreover a 'jealous' wife (highlighting the sexual grounding of her mother's decision), *over* her identity as a mother. The implication of that decision is made clear in Fraser's conclusion that her mother was 'a flawed mother' who failed to protect her.

As we saw in Chapter 5, however, when a person is categorized in a certain way, it is possible that others who want to challenge the interpretation bestowed upon a particular act or event can use the very same categorization in order to produce an alternative interpretation. In this case, for example, a feminist reader may object to the fact that Fraser uses the category 'jealous wife' as a means of explaining why Sylvia's mother failed to protect her. It could be argued that this perspective presents a 'distorted' and patriarchal view of the mother's situation. The negative judgment of the mother, potentiated by the description of her as a 'jealous wife', can be discredited by challenging some of the assumptions embedded within this description. For example, it is clear that Fraser, by emphasizing her mother's 'jealous wife' status, points towards her mother's supposed inner 'desires' and 'needs'. This is made clear in her rhetorical question: 'Did some of the wronged and jealous wife *in you* respond to the gall of that?' (i.e. the fact that Sylvia was sleeping with her father at the age of five). This focus upon inner psychological conflict as providing the 'reason' for the mother's failure to act can be challenged by adopting an alternative perspective. This perspective would locate the 'reason' for the mother's failure to act within the social and historical context, by highlighting some of the factors impinging on the mother's ability to protect her child.

For example, it could be pointed out that Sylvia Fraser was being abused in the 1940s/50s. These years were portrayed in Friedan's *The Feminine Mystique* (1965). In this book, Friedan highlights the fact that ideal female behaviour in the 1940s/50s consisted of a glorification of domesticity and passivity. Popular magazines upheld and cherished the receptivity and passivity of women's sexual nature. A woman's vocation was her husband, her home and her family. The period was marked by a new conservatism creeping into the national consciousness with a strong desire to return to the hearth, and an American postwar craving for 'Mom and apple pie'. Remedies for women's discontent included recommendations such as the following made by Deutsche in her two-volume *The Psychology of Woman: A Psychoanalytic Interpretation*:

> ... To relinquish any goals of her own and to identify and fulfil herself through the activities and goals of [her] husband. ... The daughter should devote her life to her father and thus make a satisfactory sublimation. ... (Deutsche, cited in Hewlett, 1987, p. 159)

In the film *The Tender Trap* (1955), the actress Debbie Reynolds sums up the whole situation when she asks: 'Don't you think that a man is the most important thing in the world? A woman isn't a woman until she's married and had children.' In addition to these historical factors, it is also important to take account of social factors such as the isolation of motherhood and the economic dependency of women on men (a predominant theme in the first section of *My Father's House* – see Chapter 4). Even if the mother had been able to convince authorities that her child was being abused, where would she have gone to, and how would she have brought up two children with no means of economic support?[1]

It is in anticipation of criticisms regarding her failure to take into account such considerations that Fraser provides a brief rendition of the historical and social circumstances in which her mother lived. After having concluded that her mother was a 'flawed mother' who failed to protect her, the reader is then confronted by a 'look again' procedure. This procedure involves the introduction of a social and historical dimension for assessing the mother's failure to protect. For example, Fraser comments that when her mother was born at the turn of the century, girls who did not marry were dismissed as spinsters. Moreover, war and depression delayed courtship and Sylvia's mother married her father because he had what was considered to be 'a good job'. Divorce was out of the question because of religious, moral and economic considerations. Fraser concludes that it was through such conventions that her mother acquired her 'lot in life'.

Initially, I interpreted these brief comments as attempts to mitigate the mother's responsibility for her failure to protect her child, by appealing to environmental factors beyond her control. It soon became clear, however, that this was not the case at all. After having listed a number of social and historical factors, Fraser then proceeds to argue in the following way: '*Thus* you elected to stay at your post, to refuse to see what was there to be seen . . .' (p. 232). Here, it is clear that consideration of these factors does not serve to 'excuse' the mother for her failure to protect. Rather, it serves to provide *further grounds* to account for her mother's failure to protect, by pointing to the potentially harmful consequences (such as stigmatization), that may have been forthcoming if she had chosen an alternative course of action. In this way, the mother's failure to protect appears as a 'motivated decision'. Hence, the net effect of considering the impact of social and historical factors on the mother's behaviour is to further justify Fraser's initial premise, i.e. the fact that the mother had knowledge of the abuse 'all along'.

By using the consideration of social and historical factors as a means of justifying her own position, the author is then free to expand on her psychoanalytic interpretation of the mother's action. Hence, the reader is returned to the early years of the mother's 'personal' biography in order to find the reason for the mother's failure to act on her knowledge. The mother is characterized as seeing 'Not what *is*, but what *is seen to be*' (p. 232). She sees 'only' the 'appearance' but not the 'reality'. Here, like Sylvia when she was suffering abuse at the hands of her father, Sylvia's mother shuts off the 'reality' of the event, inventing her own reality as a means of coping with the trauma. However, Sylvia's inability to 'see' the reality of the situation was triggered by an 'original' traumatic incident (the rape scene – see Chapter 6), which occurred when she was five years old. Is there a similar 'original' scene occurring within the mother's early years which caused repression and resistance? Is it this scene that predisposes the mother to 'blindness' in her later life? Searching through the early years of her mother's life, the author locates one particular incident which leads to her mother's 'refusal' to 'see reality'. This incident occurs when the mother, as a child, finds her father hanging dead (he committed suicide) in the rafters of their farmhouse. Fraser portrays the scene as follows:

> You open the door and, yes, your father is there – hanging from the rafters, his forty-four-year-old face a strangulated mask never to be erased from your dreams. *After seeing that, how many other things would you not want to see.* (p. 233)

In this way we can see how the mother's failure to acknowledge the reality of the abuse is located in accordance with the psychoanalytic framework, i.e. within the early years of her biography.

Having drawn a comparison between the repression experienced by Sylvia and her mother owing to the impact of traumatic experiences in early childhood, it is now important to highlight a crucial distinction between the two cases. This distinction centres around the issue of knowledge and has great implications for whether or not the individual can be held responsible for his/her own actions. If we return to the very early stages of *My Father's House*, it is clear that Sylvia is characterized as having split into two because of the traumatic experiences of childhood sexual abuse which force into play the repressive forces of the unconscious. From this point onwards, not only does Sylvia fail to 'see' or 'hear' the activities performed by her 'other self', but she also has *no knowledge* of them. However, despite the fact that the mother is also portrayed as repressing knowledge of the 'primal scene' in which her father hanged himself, her situation is not directly comparable to that of Sylvia's. This is because, although Sylvia's mother is metaphorically 'blind' – and thus, like Sylvia, is unable to 'see' the reality of the abuse, this does not result in the conclusion that she has *no knowledge* of the abuse. Indeed, as my findings have shown, the author works from the assumption that the mother has always had knowledge of the abuse. The use of verbs implying decision and choice on the part of the mother all confirm this finding: 'How many other things would you not *want* to see?' (p. 233), asks Fraser; 'You *elected* to stay at your post'; 'you *refused* to see what was there to be seen' (p. 232). Moreover, this results in the conclusion:

> Yes, mother, you had much in your life you *dared* not see. So it comes to this: can I blame you for *choosing* selective sight, the same method of survival that I, your daughter, *would choose*? (p. 233)

Here, then, it is clear that a crucial distinction is maintained between Sylvia's and her mother's response. Sylvia's mother is portrayed as having chosen to repress her knowledge of the abuse. By contrast, over the course of the text Sylvia's actions are portrayed as the passive product of a relentless stream of uncontrollable forces.

The Father – Psychological Explanations

The chapter entitled *My Father* opens by portraying a scene in which Sylvia is looking at some past photographs of herself. These photographs were taken during her adolescence. Sylvia looks at herself 'in velvet formal', in 'cheerleading outfit' and in 'bathing suit'. These photographs clearly make reference to the past part of herself called 'Appearances'. Sylvia then proceeds to look at a photograph of her father when he received his gold-pin for 40 years' 'faithful service' at the Steel Company. Fraser comments that in his view, he had accomplished something through those 40 years of service. She then goes on to list his 'other moments of pride', which came about when he played for the 'Hamilton Rough Riders football team' and when he served as a lieutenant during the First World War. The platitudes offered at his funeral referred to him as 'a Christian man who didn't smoke or drink', a 'man who never took the Lord's name in vain', a 'good neighbour who … kept his snow shovelled, his leaves raked and his bills paid' (p. 239). Fraser suggests that such platitudes 'held their own truth' and she questions whether or not it is fair to dismiss 'all this' as hypocrisy? Is it not the case that her father experienced two realities: the reality that can be seen from the photographs, and the 'other' reality which does not figure in those photographs?

The narrative then proceeds to elaborate further upon the father's 'second reality'. Sylvia's father is portrayed as 'child-like' in a similar way to the author's portrayal of her own 'other self' over the course of the text. For example, he is characterized as shouting and waving his fists 'like a child in a high chair' (p. 239). Similarly, his rage, like a child's, is described as 'impotent' because although he always 'demanded and was obeyed', unfortunately, 'he was never heard' (p. 239). As we have already seen in the case of Sylvia and her mother, the themes of 'blindness' and 'deafness' point towards psychological problems of repression deriving from traumatic events occurring during the early years of childhood. Here, reference to the fact that the father was never 'heard' implies that he may also have had psychological problems dating back to his early experiences. Moreover, further references to 'acute internal problems', 'loneliness' and 'frustration', as factors causing the father to behave in the way he did, support this interpretation.

The fact that the 'second reality' indicated above refers to an 'other self' of the father analogous to the 'other self' of Sylvia, becomes most apparent when the question of what *caused* the father to have such a distorted understanding of reality is addressed. The author asks: 'Did he do to me what had been done to him?' (p. 240).[2] Was the father as 'profoundly split' as Sylvia? Was there a 'Daddy Who Knew and a Daddy Who Did Not Know?' (p. 240). Here, the perpetrator is portrayed as a victim of circumstances, a King Lear, 'more sinned against than sinning', the unfortunate product of the abuse that he too may have suffered as a child. Perhaps the most important point to note here, however, is the practical and moral implications involved in bringing forth the notion of the 'other self' at this point. As we have already seen in relation to Sylvia, the 'other self' remains unconscious. This has the implication that Sylvia's conscious self cannot be held responsible for the actions of the 'other self' because she has no knowledge of those actions. As we saw in the adultery scene (see Chapter 5), when the 'other self' is portrayed as determining the course of action, this has the effect of diminishing Sylvia's responsibility for her own actions. Clearly, then, if the father is portrayed as having a second 'other self' which he has no consciousness of, and if, in turn, it is this 'other self' which 'takes over' and perpetrates abusive acts against the child, then it follows that the father cannot be held responsible for his actions. Here, it is clear that both the victim and the perpetrator are characterized as victims.

However, in order that the pattern of the father's life does not appear too predictable or over-determined, Fraser swiftly rejoins her earlier questions with the statement that: 'I ask questions of the past but I don't expect answers' (p. 240). Of course, the idea that the author is unable to find answers about the past is mere rhetoric, and no less effective for that. The whole account, as has been shown, has consistently preserved a model of the individual as living concurrently within two realities: the 'reality' of the 'outer' superficial world on the one hand, and the 'reality' of the 'inner' psychic world on the other. It is the latter 'reality', the 'universal law of the psyche' that is characterized as possessing the key to the truth in Fraser's text. Hence, by this point within the text, the answers to the questions posed about the past consist of something of a *fait accompli*. The model of the individual developed in relation to the portrayal of Sylvia's life establishes a precedent for understanding the life and personality of her father. Hence, just as Sylvia is portrayed as suffering mental illness at later stages in her life, so too is her father.

The Question of Agency

Fraser's appeal to the notion that her father is suffering from mental illness, is, however, a claim, like any other, that is open to challenge. This is especially the case when one realizes the implications of claiming that perpetrators of sexual abuse are 'sick', or 'abnormal'. Such claims, as I have previously suggested, imply that perpetrators bear limited or no responsibility (depending upon the extent of successful mitigation) for their actions. In consequence, they may escape the penal system and alternatively enter the realm of 'treatment' and 'healing'. Their actions become 'symptoms' to be modified (see Horton, 1990).

Subsequently, an attempt may be made to subvert such an explanation of the father's behaviour by displaying his intention or *mens rea* with regard to his sexually abusive crimes. Here, we have the classic debate over whether or not the accused is 'mad' or simply 'bad'. The very same act that Fraser interprets as evidence of 'madness', 'irrationality', 'sickness' or 'perversion', that is, as an act performed without knowledge due to the impact of psychological pathology, can alternatively be interpreted as simply a morally 'bad' action.[3] Hence, critics attempting to challenge Fraser's interpretation that her father was suffering from mental illness, that he was a passive victim of circumstances, and that his actions were 'ineffective' and 'impotent', may point to other 'typical cases' of child abusers in order to invalidate Fraser's claim. For example, against the assumption that 'incest offenders' or child molesters are typically 'wimpy', 'ineffectual' or 'passive', or that their actions are 'impulsive' and not subject to conscious planning, many examples can be cited to the contrary. For example, in his *Child Pornography*, Tate (1990) provides evidence of the 'cunning' of child molesters by citing the case of David Techter, an active child molester who has abused 12 young girls, including sexually abusing his six-year-old stepdaughter. Techter records in detail his *most successful technique* for obtaining access to his victims. Such strategies include becoming friendly with parents until they allow him to take their child away on a day-trip. He states that:

> Being alone is practically the key to being able to interest them in 'extracurricular' activities. Preferably away from home so there isn't the parental figure around to reinforce their inhibitions. . . . It is also important *to make the child accept part of the responsibility 'because they allowed it to happen. . . . They take part of the responsibility themselves so they're guilty too'.* (cited in Tate, 1990)

Another example is David Sonenschein, a former sex researcher at the Kinsey Institute who has also molested pre-adolescent girls. In 1981 Sonnenschein published a pamphlet entitled *How to have Sex with Kids*. This pamphlet included points such as the following: 'Friends are a good source. Once you get to know a kid you can meet their friends'; 'It is also a good idea to get to know their parents'; 'Make sure you go from vagina to anus, not anus to vagina' (cited in Tate, 1990).

Justifying the Father's Actions

Category Pairs

Fraser anticipates the fact that her portrayal of her father is likely to be subject to criticism. Accordingly, she uses a number of strategies in order to prevent such criticism from gaining ground in the first place. Her attempts to diminish her father's responsibility by locating the motivation for his actions within a psychological reality over which he has no control are subsequently supplemented by an attempt to 'justify' his behaviour. This is clear in the author's attempt to reduce the harmful effects of her father's actions, to such an extent that she emphasizes the positive influence that the abuse may have had on her. For example, Fraser claims that in her earliest memory she is 'an infant' lying on her father's bed, being 'sexually fondled' but also being blissfully unaware of deception. She goes on to suggest that such experiences enabled her to feel 'special', like a 'chosen child'. Such a lie, she tells us, was a 'blessing' as well as a curse. It is important to note that Fraser relies on the psychoanalytic framework in order to portray the abuse in a positive light. This is evident in her description of herself as an 'infant' (suggestive of 'infantile sexuality'), and in the characterization of sexually abusive events as 'sexual fondling'. Here, then, the author justifies her father's behaviour by denying that his sexually abusive actions caused her any substantial degree of injury.

Fraser also employs another justificatory strategy associated with the 'denial of injury' strategy delineated above. This consists of an *appeal to loyalties*. Here, the author claims that her father's acts were permissible because they served as a means by which he could express his loyalty and affection for his child. Thus, Fraser makes the following statement: 'Inarticulate with pain, my father expressed his love in a perverted way which was all he could manage' (p. 241). Here, it is clear that Fraser attempts to justify her father's actions by portraying them as an 'act of love'. It is somewhat ironic that she does this by emphasizing that the 'love' relationship takes place between her father and herself as a child. I say this is ironic because, in the first instance, the 'sexual' nature of the relationship between Sylvia and her father leads us to see the relationship as 'deviant' and as a breach of social and moral norms. Indeed, as Jayussi (1984) argues, it is a fact that in cases of child abuse the moral breach is intensified when the abuse takes place between 'parent' and 'child'. In support of this claim, Jayussi discusses a case in which the defendant had attempted to throw his child into a furnace. She goes on to suggest that:

To throw one's baby into a burning furnace, when one is expected to love that child in the first place or at least to discharge one's responsibility of caring and providing for him, may be seen to be a very great moral breach indeed. (Jayussi, 1984, p. 182)

In cases of child *sexual* abuse, however, the situation is somewhat more complex. It is a typical feature of such cases, as is clear in *My Father's House*, that 'love' can be invoked as a means of justifying the father's actions. This is because 'love' is a feature which is conventionally bound to the relational pair 'father–child' and, relatedly, to the MCD 'Family' from which this relational pair derives.[4]

It should be clear from this analysis that one of the reasons why it is necessary to study how people are categorized (either separately or in relation to one another) is because such procedures are of extreme importance for the way in which we assign 'motives' to both ourselves and to other people. For example, Sylvia's father's actions are portrayed as being motivated by 'love' on the basis of the fact that he is her father. This suggests that just as certain activities may be bound to certain categories (e.g. 'protective' activity is tied to the category 'mother'), then so too are certain motives tied to certain categories (e.g. the motive 'love' is tied to the category 'father'). Moreover, just as certain activities which are 'bound' to MCDs (such as 'sticking together' is tied to the MCD 'Family') 'travel across' into relational pairs belonging to that device (e.g. 'brother' and 'sister' are expected to 'stick together'), then so too do category-bound motives 'travel across' relational pairs. This means that if the father is motivated by love, then so also is his counterpart in the relational pair, for example, his 'son' or his 'daughter'. It is clear that this 'travelling across' of motives takes place in *My Father's House*. For example, in this chapter, the problem under discussion is originally characterized as a problem 'belonging' to the father – that is, it relates to his 'internal', psychological problems. However, after having portrayed her father's acts as being motivated by 'love', Fraser is obliged to re-cast the problem as a 'two-party' affair – as a shared problem. This is evident in Fraser's statement that she 'shared a house and a crime with her father' (p. 24). Thus, it is not only the case that the father expressed his love for his daughter in a perverted way, but it is also the case that the daughter (owing to her own psychological problems) expressed her love for her father in a non-conventional fashion. The author comments that: 'The force with which I came to hate my father was a measure of the love I and my other self once bore him' (p. 241). Hence, it is not only the father who is 'guilty' of the incestuous crime, but also the daughter. This fact is made explicit in the following comment made by the author: 'He served his sentence as I have served mine, but his was for life, whereas I got off after forty-seven years for reasonably good behaviour' (p. 241).

The force of the moral expectations emanating from the way in which we categorize people is also apparent in Fraser's concern to diminish her father's responsibility for his behaviour and, relatedly, to forgive him. There is a sense in which Fraser *has* to forgive her father. This is because, as she is relationally bound to her father, any condemnation of his actions also reflects back in a negative fashion not only upon the author herself, but also upon the rest of her family. Accordingly, the father can be seen as *representative* of the family as a whole. Thus, in a somewhat ironic sense, Fraser's inability to forgive her father could result in an act of self-betrayal. It is for this reason that Fraser claims that she has to forgive her father in order that she can forgive herself and, also, that she forgives her father because she loves him.

It is possible to gain further insight into the way in which 'motives' are bound to certain categories by playing around with the use of different categories and different motives. For example, if an adult, male stranger, as opposed to Sylvia's father, had 'sexually fondled' her, would it be appropriate or acceptable to characterize the stranger's behaviour as an act motivated by 'love'? I suggest that in the absence of conventional features associated with the father–child relationship, such a characterization would be considered inappropriate. Indeed, we have a contemporary example of this issue. Associations such as the NAMBLA (North American Boy Love Association) have attempted to define the rights of adult men to abuse male children on the grounds that they are motivated by 'love' and not 'lust' (Tate, 1990). In general, however, the public response has been one of disgust and outrage. This is in contrast with the more acceptable suggestion that fathers may be motivated by 'love' in the 'sexual relationships' that they have with their children. Hence, it is possible to see that the act of 'sexually fondling' one's own child is quite different from the act of 'sexually molesting' or 'sexually abusing' *any* child. Indeed, it is important to note that the very way in which abusive acts are described, e.g. 'sexual fondling', 'sexual molestation' or 'sexual abuse', changes in accordance with *who is* doing the abusing, and who is being abused.

Universalization

Above, I pointed to a number of ways in which Fraser undercuts the suggestion that her father consciously intended to commit a harmful act against his child. These strategies involved highlighting the positive aspects of his actions, thus characterizing sexually abusive acts as being motivated by 'love', and as two-party acts for which the father cannot be held solely responsible. Other strategies are also used to deny the fact that the father consciously intended to harm the child. An interesting technique is apparent in the following statement made by Fraser: 'Though I shared a house and a crime with my father, I scarcely knew the man.... This I do know: my father was not a monster...' (p. 240). This statement makes use of what Sacks (1989) called a 'modifier'. A modifier can be characterized as follows. Basically, as we have already seen, whenever we use a certain category to describe or characterize a person, we implicitly refer to a whole range of common-sense assumptions associated with that category (e.g. the category 'child' implies innocence, naïvety, curiosity, etc.). The modifier, however, is used to highlight the fact that what can be said about any other member of a specific category *cannot* be said about this particular member (e.g. *this* child is certainly not innocent). In the above quote it is clear that Fraser draws on common-sense assumptions about men who sexually abuse children, that is, that they are 'monstrous', 'inhumane', 'cruel' and 'wicked'. However, her use of the modifier suggests that such a characterization cannot be applied to her own father: 'This I do know: my father was not a monster'. Fraser further modifies her father's status by drawing a distinction between superficial 'appearances' on the one hand, and the underlying reality on the other. This is apparent in the distinction drawn between the crime performed by 'my father', and 'the man' *behind* that crime. Thus, although we may possibly infer from the father's actions that he was a 'bad' father, this does not necessarily imply that he was a 'bad' *man*.

The distinction drawn between 'public' reality ('the crime' committed by the father) and 'private', internal reality ('the man' himself), enables Fraser to point towards a 'further layer of knowledge which, if only it were known, would throw light upon the reality of the situation. However, owing to the fact that Sylvia's father is dead, this 'underlying reality' will forever remain an enigmatic mystery. Thus, according to Fraser: 'Mine is not a story of the boot, but of the *imprint of the boot* on flesh: *imprinting*' (p. 240). All we have is the 'appearance', not the 'reality'. We do not have the 'full story'; that 'belongs' to *the man* in question.

Despite the fact that Fraser claims that she cannot fully understand her father's actions, however, she is still able to 'pity' and 'forgive' him. The author is able to empathize with her father by viewing his problems in the context of 'humanity' at large – in other words, by 'universalizing' his problems. This is evident in Fraser's assertion that: 'We are all each other's surrogates. All of us are born into the second act of a tragedy in progress . . .' (p. 241). Here, the use of vague, inclusionary possessive pronouns such as 'we', 'all' and 'us' evokes an image of 'the human race' and 'humanity'. All people, the whole of the human race, 'me', 'you', indeed 'everyone', is confounded by the same problem. The most important point to note about such vague and generic allusions to the human race is that they serve to *close* the search for an explanation as to 'why' the father engaged in sexually abusive behaviour (see Chapter 9 for further examination of such strategies). Hence, in the final instance Fraser reaches the conclusion that: 'All of us are born into the second act of a tragedy in progress . . .'. Whose fault is that? Can we blame the father for his fallibility when 'we' are 'all' subject to the same dilemma – the dilemma of humanity?

Differential Tying

Accounting for the father's actions in this way, as though he were representative of the problems faced by humanity at large, points to a rather interesting phenomenon that I call *differential category tying*. By this, I mean that there is a difference in the way in which Sylvia's and her mother's actions, on the one hand, and Sylvia's father's actions, on the other, are 'tied' into the use of certain categories used to characterize their actions. Over the course of this analysis it has become apparent that all three protagonists, at some point within the text, are portrayed as having no conscious knowledge or awareness of the abuse. This has the implication that they have no intention to engage in their various acts, and ultimately, therefore, that they cannot be held responsible for those actions. However, the important point to note here is the way in which Fraser anticipates potential criticism of the fact that the protagonists have no knowledge of the events taking place. It is in her anticipated response to such criticism that the issue of 'differential tying' becomes most apparent. For example, in the TV interview scene with Joker (see Chapter 5), I showed how Fraser's portrayal of the child victim as innocent and lacking in sexual knowledge was challenged by alterna- tively characterizing the child as a 'seductive little girl'. Characterizing the victim in this way implies that she does have the knowledge and intention to engage in sexual activities. Hence, knowledge is 'tied' or 'bound' to the category 'seductive little girl'. Similarly, the notion that the mother does not have knowledge of the abusive events is not seriously entertained. This is because her actions and motives are continuously 'tied' to the category 'mother' – a category which assumes the presence of such knowledge. Thus, it is clear that both Sylvia and her mother can be held responsible for their actions by virtue of the fact that these actions are tied to certain categories which assume knowledge of sexual activities.

By contrast, Fraser's portrayal of her father as representative of the universal condition of humanity allows her to adopt a much more philosophical and speculative perspective with regard to the question of whether or not her father had knowledge of the abuse. This is because the failure to 'tie' down his behaviour to any one category has the implication that certain types of knowledge and motive cannot simply be 'mapped onto' him in order to account for his behaviour. Hence, his case remains much more open and enigmatic, making it easier for Fraser to claim that he was not responsible for his actions. Not only does this enigmatic characterization of the father result in a reduction of his responsibility for his own actions, however, but it also reduces the possibility of considering the social and historical climate in which his actions took place. For example, 'tying' the actions of Sylvia and her mother into categories such as 'mother' and 'little girl' serves to emphasize continually the 'gendered' nature of their knowledge and activities. By contrast, the actions of the perpetrator are portrayed as seemingly disconnected from his gendered status. This means that attention is diverted away from any consideration of the impact of the patriarchal context on the father's behaviour.

Expanding on this last point, it is important to state that within this section of Fraser's text there is a notable lack of any consideration of the social and historical factors affecting the father's interaction with his daughter and family. The 'rage', 'anger' and 'love' experienced by the father are all presented as 'symptoms' of his internally disturbed psychic state. By contrast, as we have already seen in the first section of Fraser's text, such 'personal emotions' were all connected to the cultural context of patriarchy (see Chapter 4). It is perhaps pertinent at this point to recall some scenes from this stage of the text. For example, the 'love' of the child for her father was connected to her social, emotional and economic dependency upon him. Recall the father's response when the child threatens to tell her mother about the abuse: 'Your mother will do what I say' (p. 11), he tells her. He has paid for everything in his house, and therefore everything belongs to him. This gives the father the right to demand service from his wife and daughters: 'My father sits in his armchair as if it were his throne, ordering' (p. 77); 'Old King Cole and his Fiddlers Three!' (p. 77); 'the indignant demand for service: "Fetch me! fetch me! fetch me!"' (p. 114). These demands for service, in which the father expresses his 'rage' and 'anger', are clearly connected to the father's superior social and economic position as head of the household in a patriarchal society. However, the social and historical factors influencing the father's expression of his 'personal emotions' remain unconsidered in this part of the text.

Conclusion

In this chapter I have looked at some of the implications of adopting a psychoanalytical interpretation of events in order to explain certain types of behaviour. It became clear that this interpretation resulted in a number of different ways of rationalizing the activities of the mother, on the one hand, and the father, on the other. These different rationalizing strategies result, in turn, in diverse judgments regarding the knowledge, intentions and responsibility of the mother and father, respectively. For example, when Fraser brings forth psychological explanations as a means of accounting for her mother's behaviour, she does so in a way which serves to *justify* her own assumptions with regard to the fact that her mother had always known about the abuse. Hence, such psychological explanations present a picture of the mother as an active agent in her suppression of knowledge of the abuse and, thus, as responsible for failing to protect her child. But Fraser's attempt to understand the meaning of her father's behaviour, by reference to psychological forms of explanation, has a wholly different outcome. Such explanations serve as a means by which his behaviour can be *excused* because they highlight his lack of active agency and responsibility for his own actions. In the final chapter I will examine further the implications of adopting a psychoanalytical model of interpretation, by focusing upon the way in which it used to explain the behaviour of the victim herself.

Notes

1.   The ability to convince authorities in the 1940s/50s would have been highly unlikely. Even in the contemporary climate where the issue of child sexual abuse is high on the agenda of public concern, the difficulty of proving that abuse is taking place, or has taken place in the past, is well known. We only need to look at the problems of 'evidence' encountered in recent 'scandals' such as Cleveland, Rochdale, Orkney, etc. Imagine, then, the potential response of the police to a mother in the 1950s, when the issue was scarcely recognized. A mother writing to a magazine column 'Dear Abby' in the 1950s highlights the reality of the situation:

> I wrote to you several months ago about a male relative molesting my three year old daughter. . . . We confronted him and he denied everything. 'She

makes up stories', he said. Abby, how can a three year old make up stories of this kind? . . . I talked to the police and was told that you cannot accuse someone of molesting without proof. . . . 'Will they take the word of a three year old against that of a grown man who is admired and respected by all? NO! I was made to look like an *hysterical mother having hallucinations.* (cited in Ward, 1984)

2.   It is never made clear who could have been the perpetrator of such sexual abuse. According to the text, Sylvia's paternal grandfather died when his son (Sylvia's father) was very young (p. 207). Although there are continual, vague references to incest as a family trait, this is never elaborated upon in any detail. There is a repeated allusion to an 'incestuous relationship' between Sylvia's father and his sister (Aunt Estelle). However, it appears that Sylvia's father and Aunt Estelle were around the same age. This, I would argue, consists of a rather different scenario from that of sexual abuse taking place between a five-year-old child and an adult male.

3.   There are some striking examples of this dilemma within Dostoevsky's novels. For example, in *The Idiot*, General Yepanchin and Prince Myshkin discuss the beautiful Natasya Filippovna and the former claims:

> . . . I don't believe in her insanity. She's a preposterous woman, I grant you that, but, believe me, she's a deep one and far from mad. Her outburst about Kapiton Alexeyevich to-day proves it . . . it was all done for a special purpose of her own. (Dostoevsky, 1955, p. 369).

And in a later scene, as Ippolit discusses with Ganya the mental state of the latter's father:

> I'm afraid I cannot quite agree with you that your father has gone out of his mind. . . . On the contrary, it seems to be that, if anything, he's been saner than ever of late . . . he's become so careful, so meticulous, weighing up every word, trying to get to the bottom of everything . . .'. (Dostoevsky, 1955, p. 484).

One way of challenging claims to insanity, therefore, is to highlight the presence of intention and purpose either prior to the act or when the act is actually being performed.

4.   In one study of child molesters' non-sexual reasons for abusing children, reasons such as 'offering help and understanding' and 'sharing love' were given (Tate, 1990), and another study of fathers' reasons for abusing their daughters included 'giving her sexual education' and a 'need to teach her the facts of life' (Weiner, 1962). When one woman who had been sexually abused from the age of five by her father started going out on dates, her father accused her of being a whore. '"I asked him why I suddenly became a whore . . . when he'd been fucking me for years! . . . He said with him it was different because *he loved me, it was in the family*"' (Pheterson, 1988, p. 222).

Chapter 8

Apologia

... now, more often than not, psychoanalysis gives the appearance of a salvation ethic, in which, according to the Menningers,
for example, any kind of unhappiness is worth eradicating, even
if the result is bland social conformity or a Polyannic indifference
to one's own or one's neighbours' situation. (Louch, 1966,
pp. 92–3)

In fact I've reached the stage when I look at people and say – he
or she, they are whole at all because they've chosen to block off
at this stage or that. People stay sane by blocking off, by limiting
themselves. (Lessing, *The Golden Notebook* 1989, p. 413)

Introduction

Over the course of this book I have attempted to examine some of the
ways in which Fraser produces an authoritative interpretation of her
experience of childhood sexual abuse in her autobiography, *My Father's
House*. One of the central textual devices used within this text as a means
of establishing authority is the 'formulation'. In Chapter 3 I outlined the
fact that the formulation consists of a means by which the author can
continually make explicit the meaning of his/her text. In the process of
so doing, the author may aim to preserve certain meanings, to delete or
evade others and, finally, this may lead to the transformation of the
overall meaning and significance of the text. In Chapter 3, we observed
that formulations may occur on a number of textual 'levels'. These were
the 'levels' of 'utterance by utterance', 'topic/theme' and 'overall structure'. So far in this analysis I have identified how formulations work in
My Father's House at the first two levels. First, at the 'level' of 'utterance

by utterance' or 'voices' (see Chapter 3), and second at the 'level' of 'topic' or 'theme' (see Chapters 4–7). For instance, the various 'voices' in Fraser's text provide the structure through and by which an authoritative interpretation of the meaning and significance of events can be established. For example, over the course of Chapters 4–7 we have seen how the text has preserved an image of 'inner', unconscious forces as causal in determining the course of events. By contrast, this has involved 'deleting' or evading the impact of 'outer' social and historical forces on the course of events. The upshot, or the 'transformative' effect of this, has been to present an image of these various 'psychic' and 'social' forces as separate from one another. For the purposes of this study, the important point to note is that this results in a portrayal of the 'psychic' domain as 'natural' and pre-given and, thus, as having access to a 'truth' which is untainted by social, discursive and cultural factors. Some of the practical and moral implications of this perspective were sketched in Chapter 7.

Having looked at the first two levels of formulations, it is now necessary to move on in order to examine formulations at the third level of organization – that is, at the level of 'overall structure'. I will do this by focusing upon the Postscript which provides an overall summary and characterization of the events that have taken place within *My Father's House*. Here, it will become clear that Fraser maintains her authoritative interpretation of events, preserving and deleting themes in accordance with that interpretation. Finally, we address the 'transformative effect' of the healing discourse, specifically with regard to *My Father's House*, and also in relation to the experience of childhood sexual abuse more generally.

Preserving the 'Private'/'Public' Divide

At the beginning of the Postscript, Fraser seems to break away from her emphasis on 'private biography' – an emphasis that has provided the main focus of the second and third sections of the text. Here, as we have seen, there has been scant reference to 'public' chronology (i.e. dates, times, years). Now, however, as Fraser has gone through the step-by-step process of healing and returned to mental health, she has also returned to the 'public' calendar, or, in Sacks's terms, to the use of 'everybody's calendar' (Sacks, 1989, p. 86). This means that Fraser can now return to earlier stages within the text in order to 'paper over' or to clarify any gaps that remain. For example, Fraser now returns to discuss the topic of her marital break-up and her subsequent divorce. This issue has not been addressed for a long time within the text owing to the more pressing 'needs' of the unconscious. Now, however, the date of the divorce is specified. The divorce was uncontested and took place in 1977 on the grounds of Sylvia's desertion.

Other 'loose ends' also need to be dealt with. Fraser specifies the time period in which *My Father's House* was written. She tells us that it was 'three years ago', towards the end of 1984, when she decided to 'retreat' to a place where she could heal and integrate, and perhaps write a book.[1] Fraser then reports news of her ex-husband's death in 1987. The narrative then proceeds to use the present tense, indicating that this is the current reality experienced by the author.

The incident of Danny's death is used as a means of foregrounding the theme of 'Appearance'/'Reality' that has been ongoing throughout the whole text. As Sylvia examines the 'mock-up' of Danny's dead body, she reaches the conclusion that his corpse is the 'best advertisement' for 'something more' that she has ever seen. Since her college days, Fraser tells us, she has acquired more patience with the mysterious and more reverence for the unknown. Danny is no longer present, she tells us. The corpse simply contains his 'remains' – 'that which is leftover'. Danny is dead but he has also '*gone*' – he has 'risen' (p. 247). In this passage, Fraser builds upon her notion that there is an underlying, mysterious, psychic reality; an inner soul that leaves the body – the mere, material physical substrate – when the individual dies. It is, supposedly, this 'something more' which possesses the key to the 'truth' of Fraser's own life and, likewise, to the 'truth' of her father's life (see Chapter 7).

Fraser's purpose in highlighting the distinction between 'mind' and 'body' and 'inner' and 'outer' at this stage within the text becomes clear when she discusses the means by which loss can be overcome. The only way in which we can overcome loss, she tells us, is to absorb the 'good qualities' of the lost person or object. Surely, she speculates, this is the meaning of the Eucharist: 'This is my body, this is my blood'. Here, however, Fraser's reference to her loss does not simply refer to her loss of Danny through his death, but also to the loss of their marriage. Sylvia copes with this loss by focusing upon her 'good' memories of 'our twenty years of intimacy' (p. 247). In addition, in Chapter 7, it was clear that when Sylvia lost her father through his death, this paved the way for her recognition of his 'good' qualities. It is also important, however, to note that there has been another loss, another death, which I have not yet mentioned. This is the death of the 'other self' which is reported at the end of the chapter, *My Father*. In this scene, the 'other self' makes an appearance as a 'ragamuffin in a tattered sunsuit'. Fraser's healed and adult self holds out her hand to this ragamuffin – a gesture symbolizing acceptance, and then allows her to 'melt' into her chest. This results in

Fraser's assertion that both her father and her 'other self' are, at last, dead, and laid to rest. As I have already suggested, in the last chapter we saw how the loss of the father enabled Fraser to 'absorb' his 'good qualities'. Shortly, I will go on to demonstrate how the loss of the 'other self' similarly enables Fraser to absorb her 'good qualities'. Perhaps more importantly, however, I will discuss some of the wider implications that this has for the portrayal of the victim within *My Father's House*.

The Internalization of Guilt and Responsibility

When Fraser looks back over her life as a whole, she sees that life as being divided into two opposing camps. From one vantage point, Fraser tells us, she sees nothing but devastation. This is the dark side of her life, the story that she has told in *My Father's House*. However, 'like the moon', her life has another side, a side 'with some luminosity'. The dark side is the story of early loss – the loss of innocence, childhood, love, magic and illusion. It is the side which enjoyed access to the 'secrets' of the 'other self'; the side which corrupts the child's innocence by having sexual knowledge. Here is the 'seductive little girl' referred to by Joker in Chapter 5; the little girl who challenges the claim that the sexually abused child is passive and innocent – indeed, who challenges the claim that the 'victim' is a victim at all. However, as we have just seen, with the completion of the 'healing process', Sylvia's 'other self' and the recriminating sexual knowledge that she possesses has been allowed to 'die'. This death not only enables Fraser to get rid of the child's 'badness' (i.e. her sexual knowledge), but also to embrace her 'good qualities'. Such qualities are emphasized by portraying the 'other self' as '*a good child, a wise child*, as *all children* are' (p. 242). Here, reference to the fact that 'all children' are 'good' and 'wise' performs a similar function to the statement 'All of us are born into the second act of a tragedy in progress' found in the last chapter when Fraser was trying to explain the reasons for her father's behaviour. Such generalized statements serve to cut off the search for an explanation and to leave us content with a rhetorical flourish.

However, despite Fraser's claim that all children are good and wise, at a later stage within the Postscript she is concerned to emphasize the fact that 'the guilty child was me, though I didn't know of her existence. Her actions were mine for which I must assume responsibility' (p. 252). There are numerous contradictions here. How is it possible to be a guilty child if all children are good and wise? How is it possible to accept responsibility for the actions of a person of whom one has no knowledge? Nevertheless, despite such literal contradictions, the important point to note about this statement is the practical role that it plays in Fraser's 'testimony'. Here, Fraser is concerned to display her *willingness* to accept responsibility for her past actions. In doing so she uses what has been called a 'technique of neutralisation' (Scott and Lyman, 1968). This refers to a technique often used in confessions in which the 'offender' condemns his/her own actions in order to demonstrate his/her willingness to accept the moral order. It is through the use of such techniques that the Postscript takes on the tone of an apology. By acting in a way which highlights her 'basic moral decency', that is, by acting in accordance with basic social values, Fraser orientates to the possibility of receiving a more favourable decision from her audience. This is apparent through her use of mental imperatives such as 'I *must*' in the form of 'I must accept responsibility', meaning that she is morally obliged to do so.

Fraser's acceptance of certain moral obligations and responsibilities, however, also enables her to make claims to certain rights and entitlements. On numerous occasions, Fraser implies that her move towards wholeness and health consists of a moral 'right'. For example, when Fraser prepares to tell her mother about the abuse, she justifies her actions by claiming that she 'needs' a chance to be free, and, in turn, that she has '*earned* her *right*' to such freedom. The possibility of 'healing' is therefore couched in moral terms; in terms of the extent to which Fraser can be seen as innocent or blameworthy. But what exactly does Fraser's *right* to healing, and thus to freedom, consist of? How has Fraser displayed her 'earning' of that right? On what basis does she claim her *entitlement* to healing? To some extent this 'right' is connected with Fraser's move towards independent adulthood and maturity. As Fraser grows older she 'naturally' becomes wiser. It is often assumed that an older person, because of the impact of life experience, is eligible to express his/her views on the purpose and meaning of life. Indeed, *My Father's House* has been characterized as a 'beautiful and lyrical story of one woman's coming of age'. Accordingly, Fraser's 'older' and 'wiser' status is emphasized in this section of the text. As Sylvia examines Danny's corpse she takes a step back and realizes that now, 'we are the elders' (p. 248). She expresses her regret that Danny never knew her 'better' and 'wiser' self. Unfortunately, it was not possible for this 'enlightened' self to develop until Sylvia had reached a 'stable and coherent state'. In order to reach this state it was necessary for Fraser to undergo a whole series of life experiences. This 'state' could not be reached prematurely or quickly; it required a whole lifetime. Indeed, it is only through the actual course of life experience that Fraser is able to appreciate her renewed state of health.

However, in addition to the 'natural' course of life experience, Fraser's *earning* of the right to healing also derives from her presentation of herself as 'morally worthy'. Because Fraser is a woman, considerations regarding her 'moral worthiness' are intrinsically tied to her 'sexual' status, by which I mean her degree of knowledge and experience regarding sexual matters. Over the whole course of her 'testimony', Fraser presents herself in accordance with the conventional ideal of a 'morally worthy' woman i.e. as *essentially* sexually inexperienced and sexually unknowledgeable. This claim may seem contradictory given that it is clear that Sylvia's 'other self' possessed a great deal of sexual knowledge and experience that would not be considered befitting of a young girl. However, as I have stressed throughout the course of my analysis, this knowledge is portrayed as inaccessible to Sylvia's consciousness. My claim that Fraser has presented herself as *essentially* sexually innocent, therefore, is based on her portrayal of the various parts of her past which she claims she did have consciousness of. When these elements of the past are examined, it is clear that Fraser presents herself as sexually innocent and inexperienced. For example, as an adolescent, Sylvia tells Danny that she 'does not put out for the guys'. Moreover, Danny believes her (see Chapter 4). Later, when Sylvia marries Danny, the fact that she is 'essentially' a virgin on her wedding night is emphasized when Fraser tells us that she has no conscious memory of the wedding night because 'sexual initiation' is the territory of her 'other self'. And finally, when Sylvia commits adultery, the narrative makes explicit the fact that she is a 'novice' and has never slept with anyone other than her husband. Hence, by displaying the fact that she is *consciously* ignorant with regard to sexual matters, the author shows that if it had not been for the unfortunate circumstances of her childhood, then her sexual innocence and, thus, her moral worthiness, would not have been in question. The compromising knowledge of the 'other self' is a product of circumstances beyond Sylvia's control. These circumstances forced her to possess illegitimate knowledge that she would not otherwise have had access to. However, in terms of the events that Sylvia does have consciousness of, and control over, she displays the type of ignorance required of a 'morally worthy' female. Such sexual ignorance proves that Fraser is essentially innocent and thus enables her to claim her entitlement to healing and freedom on this basis.

Fraser's bid for her right to healing on the basis of her sexual innocence corresponds to the legal process in which victims of rape are routinely monitored for their innocence and for the degree of that innocence. An interesting analysis of this process can be found in Maria Wowk's (1984) examination of a transcription from a murder interrogation in which a male suspect tries to redirect blame from himself onto his female victim, by portraying her in a sexually degrading manner. For example, the suspect claims that his victim propositioned him, and makes out that her behaviour was sexually explicit. By doing so, he portrays the victim as 'sluttish' and 'whorish' – a characterization which goes against our common sense knowledge of what women 'should be like' (for instance, women should be sexually 'passive' and 'wait until asked'). By describing his victim in this way, the male suspect tries to reduce her innocence and, thus, her 'right' to the independence and freedom that any morally competent citizen of the community deserves. It is precisely these types of morally degrading descriptions that Fraser tries to avoid in her presentation of herself as essentially sexually innocent.

However, it is important to note that, in the process of so doing, Fraser feeds into cultural prejudices regarding distinctions between 'good' and 'bad' women; between 'virgins' and 'whores'. This becomes most apparent when we realize that her presentation of herself as sexually innocent requires her to marginalize and 'silence' the 'other' part of herself who does possess morally inappropriate knowledge. As I have already shown, this exclusion of the 'other self' comes about when she is symbolically allowed to die. Nevertheless, such exclusionary activities carry very harmful consequences with regard to the issue of childhood sexual abuse. Researchers such as Kitzinger (1988) and Summit (1988) have recently explored these consequences in relation to society's 'ideology of innocence' regarding children. This ideology encourages us to view children as passive, innocent, sexually unknowledgeable and essentially 'good'. The problem with such an ideology, however, is that children who do not conform to such an ideal (such as children who have been sexually abused who often display signs of active sexual behaviour) may then be subject to castigation, prejudice and stigmatization. This is known in the professions dealing with childhood sexual abuse as the 'damaged goods syndrome'.

Part and parcel of Fraser's attempt to heal herself involves not only her ability to 'forgive' the 'bad' part of herself, but also her ability to forgive her father. As we saw in Chapter 7, Fraser feels that it is necessary to forgive her father because he did not actually intend to harm her; rather, his acts were really only an 'expression of love'. This 'love' could not be expressed in a 'normal' way because Sylvia's father suffered from a form of mental instability which derived from his own traumatic childhood. In this section of the text, the fact that her father's acts were motivated by 'love' is reiterated. When discussing the 'light' side of her life, Fraser tells us that she experienced unconditional love with Danny, her ex-husband. She then goes on to refer to the fact that she had been damaged 'by love' at an early age. This 'love' is the love that motivated her father to perpetrate sexual abuse upon her. It is important to note here that Fraser refers to her husband's and her father's love for her in the same breath, so to speak. This has the implication that no distinction is drawn between the two relationships, that is, between Sylvia and her husband on the one hand, and Sylvia and her father on the other. This lack of distinction is reminiscent of the first stage of Fraser's text which is influenced by the socialist feminist discourse. Here, the father's and Danny's 'love' for Sylvia were seen as part and parcel of the patriarchal context in which the importance of male ownership and possession is emphasized. However, this is not the way in which these events are now interpreted. In accordance with the psychoanalytic framework, the fact that the relationship experienced by Sylvia and her husband is *qualitatively* distinct from the 'relationship' experienced by Sylvia and her father is seen as irrelevant. From this Oedipal perspective, Fraser's 'love' for her husband is interpreted as a mere repetition of her earlier 'love' for her father. This exclusive focus upon the 'love triangle' of the unconscious life, however, fails to take into consideration the 'public' context of the various relationships. By this, I mean that the rights, duties and obligations pertaining to a father's 'love' relationship with his child are distinct from those pertaining to a husband's 'love' relationship with his wife. Most importantly, in the latter case, the two parties have entered into a contractual and *reciprocal* relationship. It cannot be said that the same reciprocity applies to the relationship between father and child. It is, therefore, clear that the direct comparison drawn between Sylvia's love for her father and husband is a product of her adoption of the psychoanalytic framework. Moreover, as Fraser's 'need' to forgive her father is based on her perception of his acts as being motivated by 'love', it can also be said that the necessity for forgiveness also stems from the psychoanalytic perspective.

However, the fact that Fraser is motivated to forgive her father, owing to the influence of the psychoanalytic perspective, has remained unnoticed. Fraser's willingness to forgive has been interpreted as a purely altruistic act, motivated by the author's virtuous personality. This is clearly apparent in reviewers' responses to *My Father's House*, some of which I reproduce below. For example, it has been claimed that Fraser displays 'a remarkable capacity for forgiveness' (Kirkus Review, 1988, p. 512); '*My Father's House* . . . is told with compassion and honesty and, surprisingly, without the blind rage one might expect' (Mackay, 1987, p. 3); 'Fraser's haunting story of incest is revealed with chilling restraint and with surprising empathy for the father who abused her' (Matthews,

1990, p. 93); and 'In a moving conclusion, Ms. Fraser grants her dead father her understanding and forgiveness . . .' (Johnston, 1988, p. 24). My point here is that Fraser's 'surprising empathy', her 'remarkable capacity for love and forgiveness' and her lack of 'blind rage' are not particularly surprising when they are viewed in context. That is to say, Fraser has undergone a lengthy period of psychotherapeutic treatment which has understandably coloured her interpretation of her past life. As many types of psychotherapeutic treatment emphasize the importance of 'forgiveness' and 'empathy' in the move towards mental health, it is not particularly remarkable that Fraser should display such capacities in her autobiography.

Disclaimer: Orientating to Criticism

In order for Fraser to forgive both herself and her father, it has been necessary for her to highlight the 'light' or the positive side of the abuse that she suffered as a child. Hence, she has characterized her 'relationship' with her father as being motivated by reciprocal 'love' on the part of both her father and her 'other self'. Although this may enable Fraser to come to terms with her past, this interpretation of events may present considerable difficulties for other victims of childhood sexual abuse. Fraser's perspective could lead to the conclusion that her father's acts were 'not so bad after all'. Moreover, the fact that Fraser has been able to cast aside her status as a victim and, thereby, has been able to adopt a more independent and responsible position within society, may also have negative implications for other victims of childhood sexual abuse. This is because Fraser provides us with evidence of the fact that 'victims' are not forever tied to their victim status. She demonstrates that there is a path which victims can take in order to 'heal' and make themselves well again. The problem here is that this can quite easily lead to the expectation that the individual victim should drop his/her victim status and move towards a 'healed' status. Moreover, in the event of a victim failing to do this, the fault can then be laid at the door of the individual for his/her failure to act upon initiative, or for his/her failure to be insufficiently motivated to change his/her situation. The main problem here is that too much emphasis is placed upon the victim's 'free will', and not enough upon the structural conditions influencing his/her capacity to exercise such freedom of choice.

Fraser is aware of the fact that she may be accused of adopting this kind of perspective. Consequently, she is concerned to distance herself from such accusations. She does this by drawing a contrast between her own relatively privileged position on the one hand, and the position of the 'average', run-of-the-mill victim of child sexual abuse, on the other. Fraser accounts for her own ability to 'heal' from abusive experiences by pointing to a number of factors. To begin with, Fraser tells us, she had an abundant amount of help from friends and healers.[2] In other words, the author makes reference to a 'circuit of agents' (Goffman, 1968, p. 126) who helped her to pass from 'victim' status to her subsequent 'healed' status. Additionally, however, she tells us that her story is a 'middle-class story' and, as such, she had access to educational and social resources which enabled her to 'fight back' and to change her situation. Initially, here, it seems as if Fraser is locating her 'personal' move towards psychological health within the context of wider social and historical factors. However, just as Fraser brought forth a consideration of such factors as a means of justifying her own (psychoanalytically influenced) assumptions regarding the mother's knowledge about the abuse, so too does she refer to social and historical conditions here, as a means of justifying her (psychoanalytically inspired) act of 'forgiving the abuser'. That is to say, Fraser suggests that it was her access to superior social and educational resources which *enabled* her to forgive her father. Not only did they enable her to do so, however, but access to such resources made her realize that it was *necessary* to forgive her father – they '*required*' her to forgive him. According to Fraser, she is 'required' to forgive because if she does not do so, her father's crime will be perpetuated. To quote Fraser:

> Children who were in some way abused, abuse others; victims become villains. Thus, not to forgive only perpetuates the crime, creates more victims. (p. 252)

This statement creates a rhetoric of inevitability. Fraser does not simply suggest that forgiving the abuser may help the victim to recover mental health. Rather, she states that the act of forgiveness is an essential requirement, a prerequisite, an imperative, an act which must be undertaken if good health is to ensue. Moreover, use of the plural 'children' in the statement 'children who were abused, abuse others', is presented as an objective fact, implying that *all* and *every* child who has been abused will, inevitably, abuse others. This is clearly not the case and such a vague generalization allows no room for a consideration of the different responses of victims of child sexual abuse. For example, an important factor to consider when examining the issue of the 'cycle' of sexual abuse is the different responses of male and female victims of child sexual abuse. Research suggests that male victims display a higher propensity to repeat the cycle of abuse than do female victims (Horton, 1990). However, given the inevitability of the perpetuation of the cycle of abuse, according to Fraser's perspective, the only realistic and responsible solution is to 'forgive' the abuser. Then, somewhat magically, it seems, the circle of victimhood will cease. There will be no more abuse. This 'health requirement' seems to solve a complex social problem with remarkable ease by turning:

> ... the fright of chaos into the comfort of the known; the burden of doubt into the pleasure of certainty; the dilemma of moral judgment into the opaque clarity of medical truth. (Reich, cited in Bloch, 1981, p. 334)

In her concern to present herself as upholding the cause of victims of child sexual abuse, however, Fraser is adamant that the 'requirement' to forgive does not make the crime of sexual abuse more acceptable. In order to expand on this point, however, Fraser is forced to draw on cases other than her own. This is because, as we have seen in Chapter 7, Fraser's forgiveness of her father *does*, undoubtedly, result in a portrayal of his crime as more acceptable than at earlier stages within the text. In drawing on cases other than her own, therefore, Fraser is able to emphasize the harmful and negative impact that childhood sexual abuse has had on many individuals. Mental institutions, prisons, hostels, shelters and addiction centres are full of persons who have been sexually abused and who have not recovered, Fraser tells us. Moreover, 'sex between an adult and a child always involves emotional and physical brutality. It is a crime that cripples, usually for life' (p. 252). Here, it is clear that Fraser anticipates the criticism that she has not paid enough attention to the negative effects of childhood sexual abuse. It is interesting to note the way in which she uses different words to describe the experiences that she herself suffered at the hands of her father, and those suffered by the unfortunate people listed above. For example, the events taking place in the above cases are described as 'sex', 'sexual abuse', and 'rape'. By contrast, from her 'healed' perspective, Fraser describes the events perpetrated upon her by her father as 'expressions of love', 'sexual fondling' and a 'sexual relationship'. This obviously has implications for the way in which we interpret the events taking place between Sylvia and her father on the one hand, and those events taking place amongst the 'other' unfortunate victims of child sexual abuse.

Re-integration, Psychological Adaptation and Closure

Having drawn a contrast between her own position as a victim, and that of other victims less fortunate than herself, Fraser proceeds to elaborate on her understanding and interpretation of life at a more general and philosophical level. As I have already suggested, the patient's move towards 'healing' and mental health involves a return into the 'normal' community, which, in turn, means that the patient must learn to accept responsibility for his/her own actions, and thus gain a certain degree of independence and self-control. Hence, the patient must display a willingness to accept the conventions and values of the community to which s/he belongs. This orientation towards community values includes a certain amount of deference; the individual must discard, or at least regard as less important, his/her egocentric aims and aspirations. In accordance with this moral requirement, Fraser renounces her earlier self-centredness. She tells us that her main regret is 'excessive self-involvement'. Too often she 'sleepwalked' through other people's lives with her 'eyes turned inward' (p. 253). Moreover, her toughest lesson was to renounce her 'own sense of specialness'. She had, instead, to learn how to see the 'specialness of the world' around her. Her 'pride of intellect' has been shattered. If she did not know about half of her own life, she asks, then what other knowledge can she trust?

Here, it is clear that Fraser extends her vision from beyond her own 'personal' sphere and demonstrates her respect for the knowledge of other people and the world around her. As the author returns to the world of 'normality', we are once more able to rely on 'public' knowledge of 'the world'. We are no longer confined to the symbolic imagery of the 'private' unconscious self. We are, rather, returned to 'everyone's' knowledge; the knowledge that is considered part of the 'social heritage' of the community to which we belong. The fact that Fraser orientates to this 'social heritage' is highlighted by her repeated use of plural first-person pronouns such as 'we', 'us' and 'ours'. As Harre and Muhlhausler (1990) point out, 'we' is most frequently used as a means of signalling group membership. Hence, when Fraser uses the pronoun 'we' she introduces and develops a bond between herself and her readers. Use of the pronoun 'us' similarly brings the author and the reader together in order to emphasize their joint enterprise. Additionally, as we saw in Chapter 7, both the pronouns 'we' and 'us' can be used to bring forth very general forms of categorization such as 'all people in general', 'the human race' and 'humanity'. For example, when Fraser was trying to seek an explanation for her father's behaviour, her use of the statement 'All of us are born into the second act of a tragedy in progress', served as a means by which she could close this search. This is because use of the pronoun 'all' generalized her father's problems into the enigmatic and mysterious problems facing the whole of humanity. A similar statement can be found in the Postscript when the author claims that: 'All of us are haunted by the failed hopes and undigested deeds of our forebears' (p. 253). Here, use of the collective pronoun 'all' serves to highlight the inextricable relationship that each individual has with the past.

This understanding of the nature of human life is expanded into a wider understanding of the nature of the universe and the forces of time and space. Fraser tells us that in place of her narrow world of cause and effect – in place of her 'rational' understanding of the world, she has burst into an 'infinite world full of wonder'. The whole mystery of the universe now has her reverence (p. 253). She now understands 'life as a journey' in which she has travelled 'from darkness into light'. 'Things do add up', speculates Fraser, 'life does have shape and maybe even purpose' (p. 253). Here, the author seems to suggest that Nature does represent some kind of order. But she preserves a notion of the mystery of that order by suggesting that its essence is unknowable to us.

For the purposes of this analysis, the most important point to note about these vague and general statements regarding the nature of individual humanity and the relationship between human beings and the universe is that they are used, as in other sections of the text, as a means of closing the search for an explanation as to why this or that event happened. Such statements serve a kind of proverbial function. Sacks spoke of their use in the following way:

> Just consider, with respect to the organization of the social world, that we're told how fantastically complex it is. How everything is buzzing, blooming confusion. How everybody is different. Etcetera.... (Sacks, 1989, p. 68)

Similarly with Fraser's claims about 'the mystery of the universe' and 'All of us', the fact that 'time is our ally ...', that 'life does have shape ...', that 'things do add up ...' and that 'we can grow wise ...'. All of these statements maximize the sense of accident, nature, fate, coincidence and chance. The individual is overawed in the face of mystery and vastness. The search for causal explanations is futile and is subsequently vanquished when one realizes that chance plays a large part in determining the course of human life. One is led to the conclusion that 'what happened, well, it happened, period'. Fraser's rhetorical statements are not open to question because they are not the kind of statements that one would doubt or ask for evidence of. As such, when such comments are used in interaction, they are very rarely challenged. This is because they appeal to common sense and to 'what is known by everyone'; as such, they represent strictly 'traditional' or 'proverbial' information about the world. Hume, for example, talked about the fact that when he was sitting and doing philosophy there were lots of things that he could doubt but as soon as he got up and walked out of his room they were just there. The kind of statements used by Fraser here refer to this realm in which our knowledge of the world is 'just there' and not open to doubt.

Fraser's use of such statements, therefore, enables her to bring her search for an explanation to a close. These remarks also enable her to bring the text as a whole to a close. By moving towards a consideration of worldly, philosophical issues, Fraser gears into the rest of the world; a world that is organized apart from the text. In the Postscript the emphasis on growing older and wiser, the thematization of life as a journey and the final focus upon the death of Sylvia's mother, who, 'her final journey completed, has run out of breath' (p. 254), serves as a means of closing the text. In this way, as Sacks pointed out, the text has a 'proper ending'. By this, he referred to the fact that we use social conventions as a means of 'closing' or 'ending' a course of interaction. For example, the day ends for a person when s/he goes to sleep. It is by implicit reference to such socially organized conventions of closure that 'the last sleep death' so often figures in the closing scenes of much Western literature.

The move towards closure in the search for explanations indicates the way in which the 'healing' solution advocates a passive adaptation and adjustment to social norms and values. Through the use of proverbial statements, Fraser displays her willingness to accept common-sense notions of what is 'good', 'natural' and morally 'right'. Fraser is no longer concerned to question or criticize the accepted moral values of society. Rather, in her return to 'normality' and mental health, she reproduces those values in her understanding of what constitutes 'natural' and 'unnatural', 'good' and 'bad' and, relatedly, 'innocence' and 'guilt'. Indeed, if she wants to be 'normal' she must adhere to moral standards and this, as Nietzsche suggests, involves acting 'in accordance with custom, to be ethical means to practice obedience towards a law or tradition established from of old' (Nietzsche, 1977, p. 75).

The ability of the 'healing discourse' to produce an adaptation to social and moral norms was also apparent in a TV interview with the author following the publication of *My Father's House*. In this interview Fraser said that she had reached a point in her life where she no longer wished to write. 'The tortured unease which penetrated her earlier, successful novels had been purged. The urge to write was gone. *She was at peace*' (cited in Bagley and King, 1990, p. 22).[3] In this way, it can be seen that the 'healing discourse' produces a radically different understanding of how to deal with the issue of childhood sexual abuse from that put forward by the earlier socialist feminist perspective. It seems that, as opposed to radically challenging and questioning the basic moral values of a society which allows childhood sexual abuse to occur on a mass scale, Fraser is content to accept these moral values as a means of achieving independence and freedom. This fact is underlined by Fraser's proposed 'resolution' to her problems in which she advocates the necessity of expressing empathy and 'love' for the perpetrator – and ultimately, of 'forgiving' him. It is only by doing this that Fraser can express 'hope' for the future:

> I also forgive my father because I love him. That is the biggest shock of all. Not only that I once loved him but that I love him even now. For hope, read love. (p. 241)

Here, Fraser speaks from her position of renewed 'emotional health'.

Conclusion

I am now back at the starting point of this study where I suggested that in recent years there has been a tendency within some forms of feminism and social science to move towards a foundational, psychological understanding of 'personal experience' and 'subjectivity'. This perspective, I argued, fails to ground 'personal experience' within a social, historical and political context. The shift that has been documented in relation to Fraser's text is a telling example of this tendency. Within the latter half of Fraser's text, the portrayal of the victim's personal experience of childhood sexual abuse is strikingly different from the portrayal of her experience in earlier parts of the narrative. Moreover, the interpretive shift encountered within Fraser's text reflects a wider historical shift in relation to treatment of the issue of child sexual abuse. Earlier accounts, which were written under the impact of feminist struggles for conceptual and political unity, produced an entirely different picture of events to that emerging in and through the 'healing' discourse. It is clear here that 'feminism's grappling with the personal as political promises to degenerate into an absorption with the personal as personal' (Cocks, 1984, p. 48).

As Kitzinger argues, the 'thriving incest industry' of the 1980s and 1990s is riddled with psychological explanations which appropriate feminist rhetoric but which dismiss feminist ways of understanding our lives (Kitzinger, 1992, p. 400). 'Psychology', she argues, 'has devised a framework for processing our "personal experiences" which erases feminist questions about the implications of sexual violence for relations between men and women . . .' (1992, p. 400). Thus, within the 'healing' discourse, emphasis is shifted away from the social and political context onto an exploration of the psychological facets of power. That is to say, the analysis of power is reduced to an analysis of the complexities of an inner psychic life. The medicalization and psychologization of sexual abuse has reduced a 'social and political issue into a matter of "diagnosis"' (Kelly, 1988, p. 14). It is, once again, victims who are construed as potentially dangerous, maladjusted and problematic owing to their psychological pathology, rather than a problem of male violence perpetuated by male economic and political power.[4] The 'incest industry' has totally relocated and anaesthetized the problem of childhood sexual abuse, and this has had, and will continue to have, major implications for the way in which the issue is treated in contemporary society. In Armstrong's words:

> We spoke of male violence and deliberately socially accepted violation. They spoke of family dysfunction. . . . We spoke of social change. They spoke of personal healing. We spoke of political battle. They spoke of our need to hug the child within. (Armstrong, 1991, p. 30)

Such anaesthetization is not confined to the 'incest industry', however. As I indicated earlier in this study, Fraser's text highlights a rather unholy alliance that has emerged between the discourse of 'healing' and that of 'radical' feminism. Initially, as Cocks (1984) points out, the radical feminist movement spoke the language of struggle, confrontation and power. This language of antagonism has, however, in recent years been replaced by images of nurturance and harmony. Radical feminism's former preoccupation with struggle, antagonism and power has come to be seen as the product of inherently male thinking. According to the more contemporary perspective, only female thought has the capacity to return humanity to mutuality and organic connection. Cocks describes this situation in the following passage:

> In moving from themes of conflict to those of harmony and wholeness, feminists have switched their sights away from

politics to the expressive domain of culture and to the intro-
spective domain of the psyche. The very word *radical* has come,
accordingly, to have something slightly off key about it. Women
who hold to principles originally labelled as such now prefer to
describe themselves as 'cultural' or 'spiritual' feminists. They
renounce distinctions between radical and conservative, seeing
such distinctions as made in a male world that feeds on
aggressive argument and combative difference. . . . (Cocks, 1984,
p. 32)

Here, then, from within the perspectives of 'healing' and 'radical'
feminism, we see an attempt to convey what could be called the
experience of 'communitas' (Turner, 1969, p. 127). Communitas means
that people are no longer seen as separated from one another, or from
nature. Communitas has an unstructured character and refers to a
general bond which exists between people, humanity and nature at
largè. Because the emphasis is on 'general' and universal character of
humankind from this perspective, 'true experience' and 'true existence'
can only occur when a person is able to rise above (to transcend) limited
social conventions. This means that, in order to experience one's 'true
nature', it is necessary to 'stand outside' the social and structural
positions that one normally occupies in the social system. 'Truth' and
'experience', therefore, are seen as 'natural', 'given' and spontaneous.
For many millenarian movements, such as 'cultural' feminism, the ability
to experience such 'spontaneous communitas' is seen as *the* end of
human endeavour. Here, the aim is to move beyond or dissolve the
norms that govern structured and institutionalized relationships. The
problem with such a perspective, however, is well expressed in the
following statement:

Life in 'structure' is filled with objective difficulties: decisions
have to be made, inclinations sacrificed to the wishes and needs
of the group. . . . Spontaneous communitas has something 'magical' about it. Subjectively there is in it a feeling of endless power.
But this power untransformed cannot readily be applied to the
organisational details of social existence. . . . Spontaneous communitas is a phase, a moment, not a permanent condition.
(Turner, 1969, pp. 139–40)

In this study, then, I have been concerned to analyse the way in which
the 'healing discourse', as it is represented in Fraser's text, is promoting
an experiential picture of childhood sexual abuse which fails to move

from communitas back to structure. This is most apparent in the way in which the notion of 'personal experience' has developed in recent years. The idea that 'personal' or psychological experience is, in some way, pre-given, natural, direct and unmediated – and, in turn, the idea that such experience has the capacity spontaneously to 'express' the truth – is endemic to the contemporary perspective on survivors' experiences of childhood sexual abuse. The practical effect of adopting such a perspective is that claims to 'personal experience' are seen as sacred; they are mystified, they are not grounded and, perforce, they cannot be challenged.

I began this study, however, with an alternative theoretical perspective – a perspective which puts forward the view that 'personal experience', 'subjectivity', 'identity' and all other 'mental' processes, as they are traditionally conceived, do not exist in a vacuum. Rather, I have argued, seemingly psychological, 'private' attributes and processes always exist within a 'public' social and cultural environment. In this book I have attempted to apply this theoretical perspective to an empirical study of one woman's reported 'personal experience' of childhood sexual abuse. Accordingly, I have been concerned to ground Fraser's 'private' experiential claims within a 'public' discursive domain. In this way it has been possible to replace Fraser's 'personal experiences' and, more specifically, the ways in which she accounts for those experiences, back into the 'public' world of language and communication. Moreover, this has the implication that her work is made accountable – that is, open to debate.

The theoretical idea that 'personal experience' and 'subjectivity' are socially constructed through the use of language and discourse within a specific cultural domain is an idea that is currently enjoying some popularity within a range of academic disciplines. I believe that my study of the way in which 'subjective' or 'personal' experiences of childhood sexual abuse are constructed through the use of different discourses within contemporary society is an important contribution to this field. I also believe, however, that this study will be of interest to those interested in, or working within the field of childhood sexual abuse. This not least because there is such a taboo involved in broaching the supposedly inviolable domain of 'personal experience' – especially in relation to the experiences of those occupying subordinate positions in society, such as adult survivors of childhood sexual abuse. However, I cannot stress strongly enough the importance of my claim that 'experiences' are not inviolable. Maintaining the assumption that they are will, in the end, result in disaster for those who are trying to make their experiences of childhood sexual abuse public. As I suggested in my introductory chapter, the issue of False Memory Syndrome is already beginning to teach us a lesson with regard to the way in which ungrounded knowledge claims are treated; they, and the persons producing them, are ridiculed and scapegoated. It is, therefore, imperative, both theoretically and practically, that knowledge claims are grounded and open to debate. If not, the isolation and closure that many victims of childhood sexual abuse experience in the context of their family homes will continue to be reiterated on a wider social scale as victims are silenced within contemporary society.

Notes

1. There are some inconsistencies in Fraser's dates here. Before retreating 'at the end of 1984' to write *My Father's House*, Fraser tells us that she 'had a strong desire to see Danny' in order to tell him about her 'discovery'. Accordingly, they met on a 'stormy afternoon in late November'. According to Fraser, eight months had gone by since her 'past had exploded into her present'. This 'explosion' refers to the reenacted rape scene when the 'story' of Sylvia's 'other self' first came to be known (see Chapter 6). However, a discrepancy arises here because in the Postscript, Fraser specifies the date of her meeting with Danny as November 1984 – eight months after the 'discovery' scene. However, according to the main text of *My Father's House*, the discovery scene occurred on an 'April afternoon in *1983*' (p. 218). This is not a trivial detail because it throws light upon the way in which 'public' chronological time is usurped by 'private' biographical time, over the course of the text. For example, the 'discovery' in April 1983 is portrayed as occurring *immediately after* the hysterectomy operation in February 1983 (p. 212), when Fraser is 'still more at home in the world of dreams than in the real world' (p. 218). This is supposedly a time at which her psychological defence mechanisms are at their lowest ebb, which *leads* to the 'explosion' of the past into the present. If, however, such an 'explosion' were to have taken place *a year* after the operation, then the emergence of the truth would appear less of a spontaneous, unmediated and direct product of the unconscious, and perhaps more a product of the psychological therapies undergone over the course of the previous ten years.
2. Note that this reference to 'healers' is one of the rare occasions on which Fraser acknowledges that the 'truth' of the past may have derived from sources other than just her personal unconscious.
3. This points to the link between mental health and story-telling (either orally or in writing). As Marcus points out, Freud implied that 'a coherent story is in some manner connected with mental health ... illness amounts at least in part to suffering from an incoherent story or an inadequate narrative account of oneself'. Conversely, at the successful completion of an analysis the patient comes into possession of her own story (Marcus, cited in Eakin, 1985, p. 170).
4. Another example of re-locating problems, unrelated to that of child sexual abuse, is 'the present penchant for talking about racism in terms of white women's guilt rather than responsibility, so that the psyche of white women rather than white–black relations becomes the focus of discussion' (Cocks, 1984, p. 49).

Appendix A

One of the most important concepts used in Harvey Sacks's work on the problem of person categorization was that of membership categories (MCs). MCs include terms such as the following: 'brother', 'daughter', 'lover', 'aunt', 'victim', 'offender', etc. MCs are ordinary terms used in the description and identification of persons. Sacks's work on 'membership category' (MC) and 'membership categorization devices' (MCDs) was introduced as follows: 'My attention shall be exclusively limited to those categories in the language in terms of which persons may be classified' (Sacks in Jayussi, 1984, p. 212). In his early work, Sacks calls the whole apparatus comprising membership categories the MIR Device. 'M' stands for membership, 'I' stands for inference-rich and 'R' stands for representative:

> That is the core of the machinery. I take it one can readily notice how absolutely central this is, for a vast amount of stuff is handled by Members in terms of the categories that it locates and the way it locates them, and the activities that those categories are used to handle. (Sacks, 1989, p. 90)

Sacks (1972a, 1972b) went on to examine some of the procedures used by people when they categorize both themselves and others. One procedure consists of what Sacks termed the 'economy rule'. This 'rule' points to the fact that it is normally considered to be adequate in conversation to use only *one* MC when referring to a person (even though there are a multitude of MCs which could characterize that person). However, whilst it may be said that the *explicit* mentioning of one category is sufficient for reference to be understood, this must be qualified by taking into consideration the fact that there is a great deal of *implicit* background knowledge informing our understanding of the meaning of various categories. I will expand on this in my analysis of 'standard relational pairs' below.

People also use other procedures such as the 'consistency rule' (Sacks, 1972a). In order to understand the force of this rule it is necessary to introduce Sacks's concept of a membership categorization device (MCD). Sacks observed:

> Frequently . . . MCs are organized by persons of the society using them, into what I shall call 'collections of membership cate-gories'. These collections constitute the natural groupings of categories, categories that members feel 'go together'. They are not constructed merely as aids to my analysis; whether or not a particular category is a member of a particular collection is, in each and every case, a matter to be decided empirically. (Sacks in Jayussi, 1984, p. 212)

MCDs are 'naturally' or conventionally organized collections of MCs. For example, the MCs 'mother', 'daughter', 'father' 'belong' to the MCD 'Family'. However, categories within one device may also be categories in other devices. For example, 'daughter' may 'belong' to both the devices 'Family' and 'Stage of life' (e.g. 'child', 'adolescent', 'adult'). It is in relation to this notion of multiple 'belongingness' that Sacks intro-duced the 'consistency rule'. Basically, this rule suggests that if two or more categories are used to categorize two or more persons, and those categories can be heard as coming from the same MCD, then they will indeed be heard in that way. Thus, in his analysis of the utterance 'The baby cried, the mommy picked it up', Sacks notes that the category 'baby' could derive from either the device 'Stage of life' or 'Family'. The Consistency Rule alerts the reader/hearer to the fact that the categoriza-tion of further persons can be drawn from one of these two devices. Hence, when the second category 'mother' is used, it is assumed by the hearer that the MCD 'Family' is relevant because this is consistent with the first category 'baby'.

In addition to the rules of 'economy' and 'consistency', Sacks specified several further properties of membership categorization. Two of these are 'inferential adequacy' and 'programmatic relevance' and these are introduced as relevant primarily in relation to what he terms 'Standardised Relational Pairs' (SRPs), a subset of MCDs (Coulter, 1991, p. 43). In this subset, the collections of categories conventionally related together have only *two* categories each, as distinct from the collections of several comprising the larger set of MCDs (Coulter, 1991, p. 43). The S-R pairs comprise groupings such as 'mother–daughter', 'father–son', 'husband–wife', 'parent–child' etc. The notion of 'programmatic relevance' as a property of the use of S-R pairs makes reference to the fact that when one part of the pair is referred to, the other part of the pair also becomes relevant. For example, when we refer to someone as a 'husband', the 'wife' part of the relational pair is implicitly brought forth. It is in this regard that we can see that the procedural convention of the 'economy rule' must be qualified. To recap, this 'rule' points to the fact that it is normally considered to be adequate in conversation to use only *one* MC when referring to a person. However, the relational pairs make clear that there is a large amount of background knowledge involved in the way in which we categorize people.

There are also variants of relational pairs such as 'Asymmetric Relational Pairs' (ARP) (see Jayussi, 1984, pp. 124–7). These refer to category pairs such as 'doctor/patient', 'judge/defendant' and 'teacher/pupil'. A characteristic feature of such pairs is that the rights and knowledge accorded to each side of the pair are not equal – hence, *asymmetric* relational pairs.

At this point it is appropriate to consider Sacks's concept of 'category bound activities' (Sacks, 1972b, p. 224). For example, 'cry' is bound to 'baby'. Here Sacks was referring to the fact that certain activities are conventionally seen to 'go with' or be 'bound to' certain MCs. This feature of category-boundedness is a very important feature of people's common-sense reasoning about their social world. In order to be classified as a category-bound activity, the activity must be such as to permit the given category to be possibly 'read off' from the reference to the activity. For example, the category 'baby' can be 'read off' from the activity 'cry'. It is also important to note that a person's failure to engage in a certain form of category-bound activity, when s/he is believed to 'belong' to a certain category, may lead to questioning regarding that person's status and membership.

Finally, some MCDs have a special property (Sacks, 1972a, 1972b), that of duplicative organization; that is, they possess a 'team-like' quality. For example, the MCD 'Family' divides the population up into members of team-like units, i.e. family units, with conventionally appropriate forms of activity such as 'sticking together', 'in-group loyalty' etc. Relational pairs of categories drawn from a duplicatively organized device can also be treated as duplicatively organized, e.g. 'father'–'daughter', and consequently in terms of 'sticking together', 'affording mutual help and support', etc. (Watson, 1983, p. 37).

Sacks's work shows how categorizations of people have, in some cases (e.g. rapist, murderer), an explicitly moral character. In other cases, the way in which we categorize people has a much more implicit moral character. Nevertheless, membership categorizations have category-tied rights and obligations that inform their practical use and the way in which people make practical and moral judgments about the social world. Categorization procedures are therefore an essential part of the way in which we organize our knowledge about ourselves, other people, and the world more generally. Moreover, our use of categorization procedures is essentially *practical*. Although we often talk generally 'about' the rights, duties and obligations that persons may or should have, it is in the course of practical, everyday encounters that rights and duties (and therefore blame, assessments, responsibilities) are organized.

Appendix B

Chapter No.	First position	Second position	
1	IV	NV	
2	IV	NV	
3	IV	NV	
4	IV	NV	
5	IV *(LS)	NV/UV	
6	IV	NV	
7	NV/IV *(A)	NV	
8	IV	NV	
9	UV *(A)	NV	
10	IV	NV	
11	IV *(LS)	NV	IV*(TT)
12	UV *(A)	NV	
13	UV *(A)	NV	
14	IV	NV	IV *(TT)
15	IV	NV	
16	IV	NV	IV *(TT)
17	IV/NV *(A)	NV	
18	IV/NV *(A)	NV	UV *(TT)
19	IV/NV *(A)		

Diagram 1 Textual positioning of voices in *My Father's House*.
Key:
IV = interpretive voice;
NV = narrative voice;
UV = unconscious voice;
*(A) = anomaly
*(LS) = lengthy stretch;
*(TT) = third turn.

This diagram displays how the interpretive voice changes its positioning within the text on a number of occasions. These include:

(a) Anomalies of the interpretive voice: These take the form of absences or a change in format of the interpretive voice. As part of the relational pair 'NV/IV' such absences or changes can be seen as a 'deviation' from the norm. In other words, they comprise a *notice-able* and *accountable* feature (Coulter, 1991, p. 45).

(b) Lengthy stretches of the IV: The length/quantity of the text produced within the IV is important because the less that is said in a conversation, or within a text, the more what is said or written is assumed to be self-evident in its meaning and implications. Conversely:

> The more that is said, the more elaboration or justification is provided, the less the appearance of transparence or self evidence. The less the elaboration there is, the more the recipient will take it that the meaning of what should be provided is obvious. (Suchman, 1987, p. 23)

The lengthy parts of the interpretive voice thus inform the analyst of the places in which the author is most concerned to justify her position, where she is most concerned to 'paper over the gaps', so to speak.

(c) Interpretive voice as third turn: Researchers who have analysed 'third turns' in speech report a number of uses such as acknowledgements, assessment, corrections and summaries (Ten Have, 1991, p. 150). Within Fraser's text third turns are used strategically. As formulations, they serve to maintain the themes established within the framework of the interpretive voice.

References

ALLEN, V. (1980) *Daddy's Girl*, Canada and USA.

ANGELOU, M. (1969) *I Know Why the Caged Bird Sings*, USA: Random House.

ANON. (1988a) 'Review of Sylvia Fraser's *My Father's House*', *Booklist*, **84**, 15 June, p. 1703.

ANON. (1988b) 'Review of Sylvia Fraser's *My Father's House*', *Kirkus Reviews*, **56**, 1 April, p. 512.

ANON. (1988c) 'Review of Sylvia Fraser's *My Father's House*', *Publisher's Weekly*, **233**, 29 April, p. 58.

APA (1980) *Diagnostic and Statistical Manual III* (DSMIII), Washington DC: American Psychiatric Association.

APA (1987) *Diagnostic and Statistical Manual III*, rev. Edn (DSMIII (R)), Washington DC: American Psychiatric Association.

ARMSTRONG, L. (1978) *Kiss Daddy Goodnight*, New York: Pocket Books.

ARMSTRONG, L. (1991) 'Surviving the incest industry', *Trouble and Strife*, **21**, pp. 29–32.

ATKINSON, M.A. (1973) *'Formulating Lifetimes' – The Normatively Ordered Properties of Some Life-cycle Properties*, MA (Econ.), unpublished thesis, Manchester University.

ATKINSON, P. (1988) 'Ethnomethodology: a critical review', *Annual Review of Sociology*, **14**, pp. 441–65.

ATKINSON, P. (1990) *The Ethnographic Imagination: Textual Construction of Reality*, London: Routledge & Kegan Paul.

AUSTIN, J.L. (1971a) 'A plea for excuses', in Lyas, C. (Ed.) *Philosophy and Linguistics*, London: Macmillan.

AUSTIN, J.L. (1971b) *How to do Things with Words*, Oxford: Oxford University Press.

BAGLEY, C. and KING, K. (1990) *Child Sexual Abuse*, London: Routledge & Kegan Paul.

BAKHTIN, M.M. (1981) *The Dialogic Imagination: Four Essays by M.M. Bakhtin*, Ed. M. Holquist, trans. C. Emerson and M. Holquist, Austin: University Texas Press.

BANN, S. (1987) 'Art', in Cohn-Sherbok, D. and Irwin, M., *Exploring Reality* pp. 83–109, London: Allen and Unwin.

BASS, E. and THORNTON, L. (Eds) (1983) *I Never Told Anyone: Writings by Women Survivors of Child Sexual Abuse*, New York: Harper and Row.

BENDER, L. and BLAU, A. (1937) 'The reaction of children to sexual relations with adults', *American Journal of Orthopsychiatry* 7, 4, pp. 500–18.

BERGER, J. (1988) *The White Bird*, London: Hogarth Press.

BITTNER, E. (1973) 'Objectivity and Realism in Sociology', in Psathas, G. (Ed.) *Phenomenological Sociology*, New York: Wiley.

BLACK, M. and COWARD, R. (1989) 'Linguistic, social and sexual relations: a review of Dale

Spender's "Man Made Language"', in Cameron, D. (Ed.) *The Feminist Critique of Language*, London: Routledge & Kegan Paul.

BLOCH, S. (1981) 'The political misuse of psychiatry in the Soviet Union', in Bloch, S. and Chodoff, P. (Eds) *Psychiatric Ethics*, pp. 322–43, Oxford: Oxford University Press.

BLOOR, D. (1976) *Knowledge and Social Imagery*, London: Routledge & Kegan Paul.

BLUM, A.F. and McHUGH, P. (1970) 'The social ascription of motives', *American Sociological Review*, **36**, pp. 98–109.

BLUMER, H. (1939) *Critiques of Research in the Social Sciences: An Appraisal of Thomas and Znaniecki's The Polish Peasant in Europe and America*, Social Science Research Council Bulletin 44.

BOGEN, D. and LYNCH, M. (1990) 'Social critique and the logic of description', *Journal of Pragmatics*, **14**, pp. 505–21.

BORGES, J.L. (1970) *Labyrinths*, Harmondsworth: Penguin.

BOURDIEU, P. (1977) *Outline of a Theory of Practice*, trans. R. Nice, Cambridge: Cambridge University Press.

BOURDIEU, P. (1992) *The Logic of Practice*, Cambridge: Polity.

BRADY, K. (1979) *Father's Days: A True Story of Incest*, New York: Dell.

BROWN, J.A.C. (1961) *Freud and the Post-Freudians*, Harmondsworth: Penguin.

BROWN, J.A.C. (1963) *Techniques of Persuasion: From Propaganda to Brainwashing*, Harmondsworth: Penguin.

BROWNMILLER, S. (1975) *Against Our Will: Men, Women and Rape*, London: Penguin.

BRUNER, J. (1987) 'Life as narrative', *Social Research*, **54**, 1, pp. 11–32.

BUTLER, J. (1990) *Gender Trouble*, USA: Routledge, Chapman Hall.

BUTTON, G. (1991) *Ethnomethodology and the Human Sciences*, Cambridge: Cambridge University Press.

CARR, D. (1986) *Time, Narrative and History*, USA: Indiana University Press.

CASTENADA, C. (1970) *The Teachings of Don Juan: A Yaqui Way of Knowledge*, Harmondsworth: Penguin.

CASTENADA, C. (1973) *A Separate Reality*, Harmondsworth: Penguin.

CASTENADA, C. (1974) *Journey to Ixtlan: The Lessons of Don Juan*, Harmondsworth: Penguin.

CAVAN, S. (1966) *Liquor Licence*, Chicago: Aldine.

CICOUREL, A.V. (1968) *The Organisation of Juvenile Justice*, New York: Wiley.

CICOUREL, A.V. (1974) *Theory and Method in a Study of Argentine Fertility*, New York: Wiley.

CICOUREL, A.V. (1985) 'Text and discourse', in *Annual Review of Anthropology*, **14**, pp. 149–85.

CICOUREL, A.V. (1987) 'The interpenetration of communicative contexts: examples from medical encounters', *Social Psychology Quarterly*, **50**, 2, pp. 217–26.

Clark, R. (1980) *Freud: The Man and the Cause*, London: Jonathan Cape and Weidenfeld and Nicolson.

COCKS, J. (1984) 'Wordless emotions: some critical reflections on radical feminism', *Politics and Society*, **13**, 1, pp. 27–57.

COHN SHERBOK, D. and IRWIN, M. (1987) *Exploring Reality*, London: Unwin Hyman.

COTTERILL, P. and LETHERBY, G. (1993) 'Weaving stories: personal auto/biographies in feminist research', *Sociology*, **27**, 1, pp. 67–81.

COULTER, J.P. (1973) *Approaches to Insanity: A Philosophical and Sociological Study*, London: Martin Robertson.

COULTER, J.P. (1975) 'The operations of mental health personnel in an urban area', PhD thesis, Faculty of Economic and Social Studies, University of Manchester.

COULTER, J.P. (1979) *The Social Construction of Mind: Studies in Ethnomethodology and Linguistic Philosophy*, London: Macmillan.

COULTER, J.P. (1983) *Re-thinking Cognitive Theory*, London: Macmillan.

COULTER, J.P. (1989) *Mind in Action*, Cambridge: Polity.

COULTER, J.P. (1991) 'Logic: ethnomethodology and the logic of language', in Button, G. *Ethnomethodology and the Human Sciences*, pp. 20–51, Cambridge: Cambridge University Press.

COX, D. (1964) *Analytical Psychology: An Introduction to the Work of C.G. Jung*, Suffolk: Chaucer Press.

CREWS, F. (1986) *Skeptical Engagements*, Oxford: Oxford University Press.

CROSSLEY, N.G. (1993a) 'The Politics of the gaze: between Foucault and Merleau-Ponty', *Human Studies*, **16**, 4.

CROSSLEY, N.G. (1993b) *The Politics of Subjectivity: Between Foucault and Merleau-Ponty*, PhD dissertation, Dept. of Sociological Studies, Sheffield University.

CROSSLEY, N.G. (1994) *The Politics of Subjectivity*, Hampshire: Avebury Press.

DALY, M. (1979) *Gyn/Ecology: the Metaethics of Radical Feminism*, Boston: Beacon Press.

DAVIES, M.L. (1993a) 'Healing Sylvia: accounting for the textual "discovery" of unconscious knowledge', *Sociology*, **27**, 1, pp. 110–21.

DAVIES, M.L. (1993b) 'Family romance: the textual production of sexually abusive love', presentation at *Romance Revisited* conference, 20 March 1993, Lancaster University.

DAVIES, M.L. (1993c) '*Reflexivitiy, ethnomethodology and feminism*', presentation at the 1993 BSA annual conference 'Research Imaginations', University of Essex.

DAVIES, M.L. (1994) *Healing Sylvia: A Case Study of Childhood Sexual Abuse and Personality Disorder*, PhD dissertation, School of Education, The Open University.

DE BEAUVOIR, S. (1963) *Memoirs of a Dutiful Daughter*, Harmondsworth: Penguin.

DE BEAUVOIR, S. (1965) *The Prime of Life*, Harmondsworth: Penguin.

DE BEAUVOIR, S. (1968) *Force of Circumstance*, Harmondsworth: Penguin.

DELACOSTE, F. and ALEXANDER, P. (Eds) (1988) *Sex Work, Writings by Women in the Sex Indusry*, London: Virago.

DELACOSTE, F. and NEWMAN, F. (Eds) (1981) *Fight Back! Feminist Resistance to Male Violence*, Minnesota: Cleis Press.

DERRIDA, J. (1981) *Positions*, trans. A. Bass, Chicago: University of Chicago Press.

DERRIDA, J. (1987) *The Post Card: From Socrates to Freud and Beyond*, Chicago: University of Chicago Press.

DEWS, P. (1987) *Logics of Disintegration: Post-structuralist Thought and the Claims of Critical Theory*, London: Verso.

DOSTOEVSKY, F. (1951) *Crime and Punishment*, trans D. Magarshack, Harmondsworth: Penguin.

DOSTOEVSKY, F. (1955) *The Idiot*, trans. D. Magarshack, Harmondsworth: Penguin.

DOSTOEVSKY, F. (1958) *The Brothers Karamazov*, trans. D. Magarshack, Harmondsworth: Penguin.

DOSTOEVSKY, F. (1972) *Notes From Underground*, trans. J. Coulson, Harmondsworth: Penguin.

DOSTOEVSKY, F. (1985a) *The House of the Dead*, trans. D. McDuff, Harmondsworth: Penguin.

DOSTOEVSKY, F. (1985b) *Netochka Nezvanova*, trans. J. Kentish, Harmondsworth: Penguin.

DOUGLAS, J.D. (Ed.) (1970) *Observations of Deviance*, New York: Random House.

DU BOIS, B. (1983) 'Passionate scholarship: notes on values, knowing and method in feminist social science', in Bowles, G. and Duelli Klein, R. (Eds) *Theories of Women's Studies*, London: Routledge & Kegan Paul.

DUNSTAN MARTIN, G. (1990) *Shadows in the Cave: Mapping the Conscious Universe*, London: Arkana, Penguin.

DURING, S. (1992) *Foucault and Literature: Towards a Genealogy of Writing*, London: Routledge.

DWORKIN, A. (1987) *Intercourse*, London: Secker and Warburg.

EAKIN, P.J. (1985) *Fictions in Autobiography: Studies in the Art of Self-Invention*, New Jersey: Princeton University Press.

ELIAS, N. (1978) *The Civilising Process*, trans. Edmund Jephcott, New York: Urizen Press.

ELIAS, N. (1992) *Time: An Essay*, Oxford: Blackwell.

FAIRCLOUGH, N. (1989) *Language and Power*, London: Longman.

FAIRCLOUGH, N. (1993) 'Critical discourse analysis and the marketisation of public discourse: the universities', *Discourse and Society*, **4**, 2, pp. 133–68.

FINNEY, L. (1990) *Reach for the Rainbow: Advanced Healing for Survivors of Sexual Abuse*, Malibu, CA: Changes Publishing.

FOUCAULT, M. (1965) *Madness and Civilisation: A History of Insanity in the Age of Reason*, trans. R. Howard, New York: Random House.

FOUCAULT, M. (1970) *The Order of Things: An Archaeology of the Human Sciences*, London: Tavistock.

FOUCAULT, M. (1973) *The Birth of the Clinic: An Archaeology of Medical Perception*, London: Tavistock.

FOUCAULT, M. (1977) *Discipline and Punish: The Birth of the Prison*, London: Allen Lane.

FOUCAULT, M. (1980) *The History of Sexuality*, Vol. 1: *An Introduction*, trans. R. Hurley, New York: Vintage Books.

FOUCAULT, M. (1985) *The History of Sexuality*, Vol. 2: *The Use of Pleasure*, trans. R. Hurley, New York: Vintage Books.

FOUCAULT, M. (1988) *The History of Sexuality*, Vol. 3: *The Care of the Self*, trans. R. Hurley, New York: Pantheon.

FOWLES, J. (1971) *The French Lieutenant's Woman*, London: Panther.

FRASER, S. (1972) *Pandora*, London: Pandora Press.

FRASER, S. (1989) *My Father's House – A Memoir of Incest and of Healing*, London: Virago.

FRENCH, M. (1985) *Beyond Power: On Women, Men and Morals*, New York: Summit.

FRENCH, M. (1987) *Her Mother's Daughter*, New York: Summit.

FREUD, S. (1896) 'Aeitiology of Hysteria', read before the Society for Psychiatry and Neurology, Vienna, April 21, reproduced in Masson, J.M. (1984).

FREUD, S. (1914) 'Remembering, repeating and working through', *The Standard Edition of the Complete Psychological Works of Sigmund Freud*, (1956) Vol. 12, pp. 145–46, London: Hogarth, New York: Macmillan.

FRIEDAN, B. (1965) *The Feminine Mystique*, Harmondsworth: Penguin.

GARFINKEL, H. (1956) 'Conditions of successful degradation ceremonies', *American Journal of Sociology*, **LXI**, pp. 420–4.

GARFINKEL, H. (1967/1984) *Studies in Ethnomethodology*, Cambridge: Polity.

GARFINKEL, H. (1986) *Ethnomethodological Studies of Work*, London: Routledge & Kegan Paul.

GARFINKEL, H. (1991) 'Respecification: evidence for locally produced, naturally account-able phenomena of order, logic, reason, meaning, method, etc. in and as of the esssential haecceity of immortal ordinary society (I) – an announcement of studies', in Button, G. (Ed.) *Ethnomethodology and the Human Sciences*, pp. 10–20, Cambridge: Cambridge University Press.

GARFINKEL, H. and SACKS, H. (1970) 'On formal structures and practical actions', in McKinney, J.C. and Tiryakian, E. (Eds) *Theoretical Sociology: Perspectives and Development*, pp. 338–66, New York: Appleton-Century-Crofts.

GARFINKEL, H. and WILEY, N. (1980) Transcribed, unpublished conversation, Sociology Dept., UCLA, 30 March.

GARFINKEL, H., LIVINGSTON, E. and LYNCH, M. (1981) 'The work of a discovering science construed with materials from the optically discovered pulsar', *Philosophy of the Social Sciences*, **11**, pp. 131–58.

GELSTHORPE, L. (1992) 'Response to Martyn Hammersley's paper 'On Feminist Method-ology', *Sociology*, **26**, 2, pp. 213–8.

GOFFMAN, E. (1968) *Asylums: Essays on the Social Situation of Mental Patients and Other Inmates*, Harmondsworth: Pelican.

GOFFMAN, E. (1981) *Forms of Talk*, Oxford: Basil Blackwell.

GRANT, J. (1987) 'I feel therefore I am: a critique of female experience as the basis for a feminist epistemology', *Women and Politics*, **3**, 7, pp. 99–114.

GRANT, J. (1993) *The Guardian*, 24 May, 1264.

GRIFFIN, S. (1982) 'The way of ideology' in Keohane, N.O., Rosaldo , M.Z. and Gelpi, B. (Eds) *Feminist Theory: A Critique of Ideology*, Chicago: Chicago University Press.

HACKING, I. (1991a) 'Two souls in one body', *Critical Inquiry*, **17**, pp. 838–67.

HACKING, I. (1991b) 'The making and moulding of child abuse', *Critical Inquiry*, **17**, Winter, pp. 253–88.

HACKING, I. (1992) 'Multiple personality disorder and its hosts', *History of the Human Sciences*, **5**, 2, pp. 3–31.

HAK, T. (1992) 'Book review: At the Will of the Body', *The DARG Newsletter*, **8**, 3, Winter.

HAMILTON, J. (1987) 'Repressing abuse: the crime against Sylvia', *Quill and Quire*, **53**, p. 33.

HAMMERSLEY, M. (1992) 'On feminist methodology', *Sociology*, **26**, 2, pp. 187–206.

HARDING, S. (1987) *Feminism and Methodology*, Bloomington: Indiana University Press.

HARRAWAY, D. (1988) 'Situated knowledges: the science question in feminism and the privilege of partial perspective', *Feminist Studies*, **14**, 3, pp. 575–99.

HARRE, R. and MUHLHAUSLER, P. (1990) *Pronouns and Persons*, Oxford: Blackwell.

HAWKESWORTH, M.E. (1989) 'Knowers, knowing and known: feminist theory and claims of truth', *Signs*, **14**, 3, pp. 533–57.

HEARN, J. (1990) 'Child abuse and men's violence', in The Violence Against Children Study Group (Eds) *Taking Child Abuse Seriously*, London: Unwin Hyman.

HEIDEGGER, M. (1962) *Being and Time*, Oxford: Blackwell.

HEKMAN, S.J. (1990) *Gender and Knowledge: Elements of a Postmodern Feminism*, Cambridge: Polity.

HELLER, A. (1984) *Everyday Life*, USA: Routledge & Kegan Paul.

HEPWORTH, B. and TURNER, D. (1982) *Confession*, London: Routledge & Kegan Paul.

HERITAGE, J.C. (1984) *Garfinkel and Ethnomethodology*, Cambridge: Polity.

HERITAGE, J.C. and WATSON, D.R. (1980) 'Aspects of the properties of formulations in natural conversations: some instances analysed', *Semiotica*, **30**, 3/4, pp. 245–62.

HEWLETT, S.A. (1987) *A Lesser Life: The Myth of Women's Liberation*, London: Michael Joseph.

HODGE, B. and McHOUL, A. (1992) 'The politics of text and commentary', *Textual Practice*, pp. 189–209.

HORTON, J. (Ed.) (1990) *The Incest Perpetrator*, London: Sage.

HUGH, M. and WOOD, H. (1975) *The Reality of Ethnomethodology*, New York: Wiley.

HUMPHREYS, L. (1970) *Tearoom Trade*, Chicago: Aldine.

HUTCHEON, L. (1984) *Narcissistic Narrative: the Metafictional Paradox*, New York: Methuen.

ISER, W. (1972) 'The reading process: a phenomonological approach', *New Literary History*, **3**, pp. 279–99.

ISER, W. (1978) *The Act of Reading: A Theory of Aesthetic Response*, Baltimore: Johns Hopkins University Press.

JALBERT, P.L. (1982) *'Structures of "News Speak": U.S. Network Television Coverage of The Lebanon War, Summer 1982'*, unpublished PhD thesis, Boston University.

JAYUSSI, L. (1984) *Categorisation and the Moral Order*, London: Routledge & Kegan Paul.

JAYUSSI, L. (1991) 'Values and moral judgement: communicative praxis as moral order', in Button, G. (Ed.) *Ethnomethodology and the Human Sciences*, pp. 227–52, Cambridge: Cambridge University Press.

JOHNSON, B. (1987) *A World of Difference*, Baltimore: Johns Hopkins University Press.

JOHNSTON, J. (1988) 'Divided against her father', *New York Times Book Review*, October, p. 24.

JONES, M.V. (1990) *Dostoevsky after Bakhtin*, Cambridge: Cambridge University Press.

KAFKA, F. (1957) *The Castle*, Harmondsworth: Penguin.
KAUFMAN, F. (1944) *The Methodology of the Social Sciences*, New Jersey: Humanities Press.
KEITEL, E. (1989) *Reading Psychosis*, Oxford: Basil Blackwell.
KELLY, L. (1988) 'From politics to pathology: the medicalisation of the impact of rape and child sexual abuse', *Radical Community Medicine*, **36**, pp. 14–8.
KENNY, A. (1975) *Wittgenstein*, Harmondsworth: Pelican.
KIRKUS REVIEWS (1988) *Review of My Father's House*, **56**, 1 April, p. 512.
KITZINGER, J. (1988) 'Child sexual abuse and the ideology of innocence', *Feminist Review*, **1**, 28.
KITZINGER, J. (1992) 'Sexual violence and compulsory heterosexuality', *Feminism and Psychology*, **2**, 3, pp. 399–418.
KUNZMAN, K. (1990) *The Healing Way: Adult Recovery from Childhood Sexual Abuse*, Centre City, MN: Hazledon.
LATOUR, B. (1988) 'The politics of explanation', in Woolgar, S. (Ed.) *Knowledge and Reflexivity: New Frontiers in the Sociology of Knowledge*, pp. 155–76, London: Sage.
LEE, J.R. (1984) 'Innocent victims and evil doers', *Women's International Studies Forum*, **7**, 1, pp. 69–73.
LEJEUNE, P. (1977) 'Autobiography in the third person', *New Literary History*, **9**, pp. 27–50.
LESSING, D. (1989) *The Golden Notebook*, London: Paladin.
LOUCH, A.R. (1966) *Explanation and Human Action*, Oxford: Blackwell.
LURY, C. (1987) 'The difference of women's writing: essays on the use of personal experience', *Studies in Sexual Politics* No. 15, Sociology Dept., University of Lancaster.
MACKAY, B. (1987) 'Review of Sylvia Fraser's My Father's House' – 'Daddy's Girl', *Books in Canada*, **16**, October, p. 3.
MALCOLM, J. (1983) 'Annals of scholarship – trouble in the archives – 1, *New Yorker*, 5 December, pp. 59–152; 'Trouble in the Archives – 2, *New Yorker*, 12 December, pp. 60–109.
MALCOLM, J. (1984) *In the Freud Archives*, London: Flamingo.
MARTIN, B. (1988) 'Lesbian identity and autobiographical difference(s)', in *Life/Lines: Theorising Women's Autobiography*, New York: Cornell University Press.
MASSON, J.M. (1984a) *The Assault on Truth*, Harmondsworth: Penguin.
MASSON, J.M. (1984b) 'The persecution and expulsion of Jeffrey Masson as performed by the Freudian Establishment and reported by Janet Malcolm of the *New Yorker*', *Mother Jones*, **9**, 10, pp. 34–7.
MATTHEWS, C.A. (1990) *Breaking Through: No Longer a Victim of Child Abuse*, USA: Albatross Books.
MAYNARD, D.W. (1991) 'The perspective-display series and the delivery and receipt of diagnostic news', in Boden, D. and Zimmerman, D.H. (Eds) *Talk and Social Structure: Studies in Ethnomethodology and Conversation Analysis*, pp. 164–95, Cambridge: Polity.
McGUIRE, M.B. (1989) 'The new spirituality: healing rituals hit the suburbs', *Psychology Today*, Jan/Feb, pp. 57–64.
McHOUL, A. (1980) 'Ethnomethodology and the position of relativist discourse', *Journal of Theory of Social Behaviour*, **11**, 2, pp. 107–26.
McHOUL, A. (1982) *Telling How Texts Talk*, London: Routledge & Kegan Paul.
McHOUL, A. (1988) 'Review article: language and the sociology of mind. A critical introduction to the work of Jeff Coulter', *Journal of Pragmatics*, **12**, pp. 339–86.
McHOUL, A. (1990) 'Critique and description: an analysis of Bogen and Lynch', *Journal of Pragmatics*, **14**, pp. 523–32.
McHUGH, P., RAFFEL, S., FOSS, D.C. and BLUM, A.F. (1974) *On the Beginning of Social Inquiry*, London: Routledge & Kegan Paul.

McKay, N.Y. (1988) 'Race, gender and cultural context in Zora Neale Hurston's *Dust Tracks on a Road*', in Brodzki, B. and Schenck, C. (Eds) *Life/Lines: Theorising Women's Autobiography*, New York: Cornell University Press.

McRobbie, A. (1982) 'The politics of feminist research: between the talk, text and action', *Feminist Review*, **12**, pp. 46–57.

Mehan, H. and Wood, H. (1975) *The Reality of Ethnomethodology*, New York: Wiley.

Merleau-Ponty, M. (1962) *Phenomenology of Perception*, trans. C. Smith, London: Routledge & Kegan Paul.

Miller, A. (1987) *The Drama of Being a Child and the Search for the True Self*, London: Virago.

Millner, M. (1988) *The Hands of the Living God: An Account of a Psychoanalytic Treatment*, London: Virago.

Mitchell, S. (1988) *Library Journal*, April 15, p. 76.

Nelson, S. (1987) *Incest – Fact and Myth*, London: Stramullion Co-op.

Nietzsche, F. (1969) *The Anti-Christ*, trans. R.J. Hollingdale, Harmondsworth: Penguin.

Nietzsche, F. (1977) 'Extracts from Human, All Too Human' in Hollingdale, R.J. *A Nietzsche Reader*, Harmondsworth: Penguin.

Okley, J. (1986) *Simone de Beauvoir*, London: Virago.

Ornstein, R.E. (1975) *The Psychology of Consciousness*, Harmondsworth: Pelican.

Orwell, G. (1954) *Nineteen Eighty-four*, Harmondsworth: Penguin.

Perakyla, A. and Bor, R. (1990) 'Interactional problems of addressing "dreaded issues" in HIV counselling', *Aids Care*, **2**, 4, pp. 325–37.

Peters, C. and Schwarz, T. (1980) *Tell me Who I am before I Die*, Middlesex, UK: Hamlyn.

Pheterson, G. (1988) 'The social consequences of unchastity', in Delacoste, F. and Alexander, P. (Eds) *Sex Work: Writings by Women in the Sex Industry*, pp. 215–31, London: Virago.

Plummer, K. (1990) 'Herbert Blumer and the life history tradition', *Symbolic Interaction*, **13**, 2, pp. 125–44.

Pollner, M. (1974) 'Mundane reasoning', *Philosophy of Social Science*, **4**, pp. 35–54.

Pollner, M. (1975) 'The very coinage of your brain: the anatomy of reality disjunctures', *Philosophy of Social Science*, **5**, pp. 411–30.

Pollner, M. (1987) *Mundane Reason*, Cambridge: Cambridge University Press.

Pollner, M. (1991) 'Left of ethnomethodology: the rise and decline of radical reflexivity', *American Sociological Review*, **56**, pp. 370–80.

Pomerantz, A. (1987) 'Descriptions in legal settings', in Button, G. and Lee, J.R. (Eds) *Talk and Social Organisation*, Clevedon, Avon: Multilingual Matters.

Poston, C. and Lisbon, K. (1989) *Reclaiming Our Lives: Adult Survivors of Incest*, Boston, MA: Little, Brown.

Potter, J. (1988) 'What is reflexive about discourse analysis?', in Woolgar, S. (Ed.) *Knowledge and Reflexivity: New Frontiers in the Sociology of Knowledge*, pp. 37–53, London: Sage.

Potter, J. and Wetherell, M. (1987) *Discourse and Social Psychology: Beyond Attitudes and Behaviour*, London: Sage.

Putnam, F.W. *et al.* (1986) 'The clinical phenomenology of multiple personality disorder: a review of 100 cases', *Journal of Clinical Psychiatry*, **47**, pp. 285–93.

Roberts, H. (Ed.) (1981) *Doing Feminist Research*, London: Routledge & Kegan Paul.

Roche, M. (1973) *Phenomenology, Language and The Social Sciences*, London: RKP.

Roth, P. (1963) *Timetables: Structuring the Passage of Time in Hospital Treatment and Other Careers*, Indianopolis, NY: Bobs-Merrill.

Ryle, G. (1949) *The Concept of Mind*, Chicago: University of Chicago Press.

Sacks, H. (1966) 'The search for help: no-one to turn to', unpublished doctoral dissertation, Dept. of Sociology, University of California at Berkeley.

Sacks, H. (1972a) 'An initial investigation of the usability of conversational data for doing sociology', in Sudnow, D. (Ed.) *Studies in Social Interaction*, New York: Free Press.

157

SACKS, H. (1972b) 'On the analyseability of stories by children', in Turner, R. (Ed.) (1974) *Ethnomethodology*, pp. 216–32, Harmondsworth: Penguin.

SACKS, H. (1984) 'On doing "being ordinary"', in Atkinson, M. and Heritage, J. *Structures of Social Action: Studies in Conversation Analysis*, pp. 413–30, Cambridge: Cambridge University Press.

SACKS, H. (1989) 'Harvey Sacks' lectures 1964–1965', edited by Gail Jefferson, *Human Studies*, **12**.

SACKS, H., SCHEGLOFF, E. and JEFFERSON, G. (1974) 'A simplest systematics for the organization of turn-taking for conversation', *Language*, **50**, pp. 696–735.

SANFORD, L.T. (1991) *Strong in the Broken Places: Overcoming the Trauma of Childhood Abuse*, London: Virago.

SARTRE, J.P. (1961) *The Age of Reason*, Harmondsworth: Penguin.

SARTRE, J.P. (1963a) *The Reprieve*, Harmondsworth: Penguin.

SARTRE, J.P. (1963b) *Iron in the Soul*, Harmondsworth: Penguin.

SAYER, P. (1989) 'Your mum and dad', *London Review of Books*, **11**, 2 February, p. 23.

SCHEGLOFF, E. (1963) 'Towards a reading of psychiatric theory', *Berkeley Journal of Sociology*, pp. 61–91.

SCHEGLOFF, E.A. (1972) 'Notes on a conversational practice: formulating place', in Sudnow, D.N. (Ed.) *Studies in Social Interaction*, pp. 75–119, New York: Free Press.

SCHEGLOFF, E.A. (1991) 'Reflections on talk and social structure', in Boden, D. and Zimmerman, D. *Talk and Social Structure: Studies in Ethnomethodology and Conversation Analysis*, pp. 44–71, Cambridge: Polity.

SCHEGLOFF, E. and SACKS, H. (1973) 'Opening up closings', in Turner, R. (Ed.) (1974) *Ethnomethodology*, pp. 233–64, Harmondsworth: Penguin.

SCHREIBER, F.R. (1973) *Sybil*, Harmondsworth: Penguin.

SCHUTZ, A. (1962) *Collected Papers I*, The Hague: Martinus Nijhoff.

SCOTT, A. (1988) 'Feminism and the seductiveness of the 'Real Event', *Feminist Review*, No. 28.

SCOTT, J.W. (1986) 'Gender: a useful category of historical analysis', *American Historical Review*, **91**, 5, pp. 1053–75.

SCOTT, J.W. (1991) 'The evidence of experience', *Critical Inquiry*, **17**, pp. 773–97.

SCOTT, M.B. and LYMAN, S.M. (1968) 'Accounts', *American Social Review*, **33**, 1, pp. 46–62.

SHARROCK, W.W. (1974) 'On owning knowledge', in Turner, R. (Ed.) *Ethnomethodology*, pp. 45–54, Harmondsworth: Penguin.

SHARROCK, W. and ANDERSON, B. (1991) 'Epistemology: professional scepticism', in Button, G. (Ed.) *Ethnomethodology and the Human Sciences*, Cambridge: Cambridge University Press.

SILVERMAN, D. (1975) *Reading Castenada: A Prologue to the Social Sciences*, London: Routledge & Kegan Paul.

SMITH, D.E. (1974) 'The social construction of documentary reality', *Sociological Inquiry*, **44**, 4, pp. 257–68.

SMITH, D.E. (1978) 'K is mentally ill: the anatomy of a factual account', *Sociology*, **12**, pp. 23–53.

SMITH, D.E. (1983) 'No-one commits suicide: textual analyses of ideological practices', *Human Studies*, **6**, pp. 309–59.

SMITH, D. (1987a) 'Women's perspectives as a critique of sociology', in Harding, S. (Ed.) *Feminism and Methodology*, Bloomington: Indiana University Press.

SMITH, D. (1987b) *The Everyday World as Problematic*, Boston: Northeastern University Press.

SMITH, D. (1990) 'The active text: a textual analysis of the social relations of public textual discourse', in Smith, D. *Texts, Facts and Femininity*, London: Routledge & Kegan Paul.

SMITH, D. (1992) 'Sociology from women's experience: a reaffirmation', *Sociological Theory*, **10**, 1.

SPEIER, M. (1969) 'The organisation of talk and socialisation practices in family household interaction', unpublished PhD dissertation, Sociology Dept., University of California at Berkeley.

SPRING, J. (1987) *Cry Hard and Swim: The Story of an Incest Survivor,* London: Virago.

STANLEY, L. and WISE, S. (1983) *Breaking Out: Feminist Consciousness and Feminist Research,* London: Routledge & Kegan Paul.

STUART, A. (1990) *The War Zone,* London: Vintage.

SUCHMAN, L.A. (1987) *Plans and Situated Actions: The Problem of Human Machine Communication,* Cambridge: Cambridge University Press.

SUDNOW, D. (1965) 'Normal crimes', *Social Problems,* **12,** Winter, pp. 255–64.

SULEIMAN, S. and CROSMAN, I. (1980) *The Reader in the Text: Essays in Audience and Interpretation,* New Jersey: Princeton University Press.

SUMMIT, R.C. (1988) 'Hidden victims, hidden pain, societal avoidance of child sexual abuse', in Wyatt, G.E. and Powell, G.J. *Lasting Effects of Child Sexual Abuse,* London: Sage.

SZASZ (1961) *The Myth of Mental Illness,* USA: Harper and Row.

TATE, T. (1990) *Child Pornography,* London: Methuen.

TEN HAVE, P. (1991) 'Talk and institution: a reconsideration of the "asymmetry" of doctor–patient interaction', in Boden, D. and Zimmerman, D. (Eds) *Talk and Social Structure: Studies in Ethnomethodology and Conversation Analysis,* pp. 93–138, Cambridge: Polity.

TURNER, V.W. (1969) *The Ritual Process: Structure and Anti-Structure,* London: Routledge & Kegan Paul.

VAN DER POST, L. (1978) *Jung and the Story of Our Time,* Harmondsworth: Penguin.

VINCENT, S. (1989) 'Courage of her victimhood', *New Statesman,* 3 March, p. 44.

WALKER, A. (1983) *The Color Purple,* London: Women's Press.

WARD, E. (1984) *Father–Daughter Rape,* London: Women's Press.

WASHINGTON, H. (1989) *Invented Lives: Narratives of Black Women 1860–1960,* London: Virago.

WATSON, D.R. (1978) 'Categorisation, authorisation and blame negotiation in conversation', *Sociology,* **12,** pp. 105–13.

WATSON, D.R. (1983) 'The presentation of victim and offender in discourse: the case of police interrogations and interviews', *Victimology,* **8,** 1/2, pp. 31–52.

WATSON, D.R. (1987) 'Interdisciplinary considerations in the analysis of proterms', in Button, G. and Lee, J.R.E. (Eds) *Talk and Social Organisation,* pp. 261–89, Clevedon, Avon: Multilingual Matters.

WATSON, D.R. (1992) 'The understanding of language use in everyday life: is there a common ground?', in Watson, G. and Seiler, R. (Eds) *Text in Context: Contributions in Ethnomethodology,* pp. 1–19, London and Beverly Hills: Sage.

WATSON, D.R (forthcoming) 'Review article: Harvey Sacks' sociology of mind in action', *Theory, Culture and Society.*

WATSON, D.R. and SHARROCK, W. (1988) 'Autonomy among social theories – the incarnation of social structures', in Fielding, N.G. (Ed.) *Actions and Structure,* London: Sage.

WATSON, G. (1987) 'Make me reflexive – but not yet: strategies for managing essential reflexivity in ethnographic discourse', *Journal of Anthropological Research,* Spring.

WATSON, G. and SEILER, R. (1992) *Text in Context,* London: Sage.

WEINER, I.B. (1962) 'Father–daughter incest', *Psychiatric Quarterly,* **36,** pp. 607–32.

WEINTRAUB, K.J. (1975) 'Autobiography and historical consciousness', *Critical Inquiry,* **1,** pp. 821–48.

WETHERELL, M. and POTTER, J. (1989) 'Narrative characters and accounting for violence', in Shotter, J. and Gergen, K. (Eds) *Texts of Identity,* London: Sage.

WIDDICOMBE, S. (1992) 'Subjectivity, power and the practice of psychology', *Theory and Psychology,* **2,** 4, pp. 487–99.

WIEDER, D.L. (1974) *Language and Social Reality*, The Hague: Mouton.

WILKINS, R. (1993) 'Taking it personally: a note on emotions and autobiography', *Sociology*, **27**, 1, pp. 93–101.

WINCH, P. (1958) *The Idea of a Social Science and Its Relation to Philosophy*, London: Routledge & Kegan Paul.

WITTGENSTEIN, L. (1953) *Philosophical Investigations*, Oxford: Basil Blackwell.

WOWK, M.T. (1984) 'Blame allocation, sex and gender in a murder interrogation', *Women's Studies International Forum*, **7**, 1, pp. 75–82.

ZIMMERMAN, D.H. and POLLNER, M. (1971) 'The everyday world as a phenomenon', in Douglas, J.D. (Ed.) *Understanding Everyday Life*, pp. 80–103, London: Routledge & Kegan Paul.

Index

Index

Index